EVALUATION OF MITIGATION STRATEGIES FOR REDUCING FORMALDEHYDE CONCENTRATIONS IN UNOCCUPIED FEDERAL EMERGENCY MANAGEMENT AGENCY-OWNED TRAVEL TRAILERS

I0482641

Michael G. Gressel, PhD, CSP
Lynn Wilder, MSHyg, CIH

Division of Environmental Hazards and Health Effects
National Center for Environmental Health
Centers for Disease Control and Prevention

December 10, 2009

Disclaimer

Mention of company names or products does not constitute endorsement by the Centers for

Disease Control and Prevention.

TABLE OF CONTENTS

LIST OF FIGURES

LIST OF TABLES

ACKNOWLEDGEMENTS

The following individuals are acknowledged for their contributions to this project: Lauren Underwood, Steve Tate, Duane O'Neil, and Phil Kuper, Science Systems and Applications, Inc. and Bruce Davis and Rodney McKellip, NASA, for their efforts to collect the data for this project; DataChem Laboratories, Inc., for providing the analytical services to analyze the air samples; Steven Emmerick, NIST, Robert Herrick, Harvard University, and Mike Apte, LBNL, for their reviews and technical input; and Larry Reed, NIOSH/CDC, Gary Noonan, NCEH/CDC and Michael McGeehin, NCEH/CDC, for their assistance with a wide variety of administrative issues.

EXECUTIVE SUMMARY

Following hurricanes Katrina and Rita in August 2005, the Federal Emergency Management Agency (FEMA) purchased more than 145,000 travel trailers, park model trailers, manufactured homes, and non-mobile pre-fabricated housing units to provide temporary housing for families who were displaced by the storms and had no other options for housing. This report contains the findings for this investigation, "Evaluation of Mitigation Strategies for Reducing Formaldehyde Concentrations in Unoccupied Federal Emergency Management Agency-Owned Travel Trailers." This research was conducted jointly by the National Center for Environmental Health (NCEH) of the Centers for Disease Control and Prevention (CDC) and the National Aeronautics and Space Administration (NASA) at NASA's John C. Stennis Space Center in Mississippi.

The primary objective of this investigation was to assess the effectiveness of a series of mitigation solutions in reducing formaldehyde concentrations in FEMA-provided travel trailers used for temporary housing following disasters. Other compounds monitored included acetic acid and 2,2,4-trimethyl-1,3-pentanediol di-isobutyrate (TMPD-DIB). Testing for other aldehydes and volatile organic compounds (VOCs) was conducted to ensure that the tested solutions were not generating other chemicals of potential health concern.

The evaluated technologies fall into four broad categories: ventilation, oxidation, diffusion/adsorption, and ionization. Sixteen different devices from these technologies (along with controls) were assessed by air sampling in 15 travel trailers before, during, and after the units operated. Researchers assessed the effectiveness of each device in reducing indoor concentrations of formaldehyde and other contaminants.

2

The travel trailers, all of the same make, model, and manufacturing date and location, each were outfitted with one of the devices. The trailers' air conditioning systems were operated to cool the trailers when necessary, and small space heaters were used when heat was required. Temperature and humidity measurements were collected inside the trailers and from a weather station monitoring ambient conditions. Air samples were collected at least twice a week (more frequently during the first several weeks of deployment of the devices). Baseline samples were collected for two weeks before and two weeks after evaluation sampling. Evaluation sampling occurred for thirteen weeks. In addition to air sampling, air exchange rate testing was performed before the initial baseline air sampling and following the final baseline air sampling.

Initially, fourteen devices were deployed for evaluation; at the approximate midpoint of the evaluation, three devices were removed from the evaluation due to ineffective performance and two additional units were added to the evaluation. One trailer served as a control. This was a pilot test that evaluated a single unit of each device (n=1); therefore, no statistical analyses were performed on the data. The performance efficiencies of the evaluated devices for reducing formaldehyde concentrations were calculated, normalizing to the control trailer and the corresponding baseline samples.

The results of the formaldehyde sampling showed that the most effective solution was a powered roof vent, which reduced formaldehyde concentrations by approximately 79%. However, the large volume of air exhausted by this device would increase energy consumption and may not allow effective control of heating and cooling by the trailers' heating and air conditioning systems. Another unit, one using a chemically treated

3

filter, was initially 77% efficient. However, its efficiency dropped steadily after the second week of service, decreasing to 39% by the final weeks of the evaluation period. Three larger prototype photocatalytic oxidation units provided were all similar in performance, with efficiencies between 50 and 55%. A replacement air conditioning system had a formaldehyde reduction efficiency of 30%. All the other tested units had efficiencies of less than 25%. Changes in temperature could have impacted the apparent effectiveness of the devices.

All acetic acid and VOC sample results were relatively low. All of the TPMD-DIB samples were below the limit of detection. Acetic acid was below applicable exposure criteria guidelines. However, it was present at levels above the odor threshold. Like formaldehyde, this compound is a mucous membrane irritant. Many different VOCs were detected, but none was at levels of health concern.

This evaluation identified several control approaches that could provide a means for reducing formaldehyde concentrations in occupied travel trailers. A ventilation solution in combination with one of the more effective air cleaning technologies could provide an acceptable approach for controlling formaldehyde exposures. The results of this evaluation are limited by its design; however, the findings do suggest that some solutions may be technically feasible, depending upon the starting concentration of formaldehyde within the travel trailer and the target concentration considered to be acceptable for the occupants.

1) INTRODUCTION

This report contains the findings for the project "Evaluation of Mitigation Strategies for Reducing Formaldehyde Concentrations in Unoccupied Federal Emergency Management Agency (FEMA)-Owned Travel Trailers." This research was conducted jointly by the National Center for Environmental Health (NCEH) of the Centers for Disease Control and Prevention (CDC) and the National Aeronautics and Space Administration (NASA) at NASA's John C. Stennis Space Center in Mississippi. This investigation assessed sixteen off-the-shelf solutions or near-market-ready prototypes for their ability to reduce formaldehyde concentrations in FEMA-owned travel trailers intended for use as temporary housing following disasters.

2) OBJECTIVES

The primary objective of this project was to assess the effectiveness of a series of mitigation solutions in reducing formaldehyde concentrations in FEMA-owned travel trailers. Other compounds monitored included acetic acid and 2,2,4-trimethyl-1,3-pentanediol di-isobutyrate (TMPD-DIB), as these were found in the air at concentrations higher than typically seen from comparative housing measured in the United States in prior work by the Lawrence Berkeley National Laboratory.[1] Sampling for other aldehydes and volatile organic compounds (VOCs) was also conducted to ensure that the tested solutions were not generating other chemicals of potential health concern.

This evaluation assessed technologies that fall into four broad categories: ventilation, oxidation, diffusion/adsorption, and ionization. Sixteen different applications of these technologies (along with controls) were assessed by sampling indoor air in closed, ventilated, and temperature-controlled trailers. All trailers were the same model, and all were manufactured on the same day at the same location. The technology test period lasted for 13 weeks. Baseline air sampling (without the technologies) occurred before and after the technology test period. Air sampling also occurred outdoors and in a trailer with no treatment technology present (study control). Effectiveness was assessed by the ability of each device to reduce the indoor concentrations of formaldehyde and other contaminants.

3) BACKGROUND

Following hurricanes Katrina and Rita in August 2005, FEMA purchased more than145,000 travel trailers, park model trailers, manufactured homes, and non-mobile pre-fabricated housing units to provide temporary housing for families who were displaced by the storms and had no other options for housing.

Travel trailers, the focus of this research, are tow-behind recreational vehicles (RVs) designed as temporary living quarters for recreation or camping.[2] FEMA-provided travel trailers included "off-the-lot" and "FEMA-spec" units. Off-the-lot travel trailers were available for sale to the general public and purchased by FEMA from RV dealers. FEMA-spec travel trailers were manufactured for FEMA following the hurricanes in 2005. FEMA-spec trailers were built with limited amenities specifically for use as temporary housing. A single model of the FEMA-spec travel trailers was used in this investigation, with a different unit being used for each technology. Fourteen units were used to test contaminant removal efficiency, and one additional unit (without mitigation equipment) served as a control.

Concerns about the indoor environmental quality of the travel trailers were initially identified in Spring 2006. At that time, several physicians reported increases in upper respiratory conditions in children living in the trailers. Since then, FEMA has become aware of the potential for poor indoor environmental quality in the trailers, specifically elevated formaldehyde concentrations in the travel trailers. The Sierra Club initially identified elevated formaldehyde concentrations in monitoring conducted inside its members' travel trailers.[3] After the Sierra Club's report, FEMA funded the U.S. Environmental Protection Agency (EPA) to conduct formaldehyde monitoring in travel

7

trailers and subsequently requested that the Agency for Toxic Substances and Disease Registry (ATSDR) review the results.[4] Elevated levels of formaldehyde were detected and ATSDR recommended "...effective interventions to reduce the levels of formaldehyde and duration of exposure and potential health effects should be identified."

Due to the concerns about poor indoor environmental quality in the trailers, the Department of Homeland Security's Office of Health Affairs asked CDC on behalf of FEMA to investigate concerns about formaldehyde in occupied FEMA-provided trailers in Louisiana and Mississippi. In December 2007 and January 2008, CDC measured formaldehyde levels in a stratified random sample of 519 FEMA-supplied occupied travel trailers, park models, and manufactured homes.[5] The study aimed to determine formaldehyde levels in occupied trailers, to determine the characteristics that could affect formaldehyde levels, and to provide information to assist FEMA in deciding whether to relocate residents from FEMA-supplied units in the Gulf Coast area. Investigators conducted a 1-hour continuous indoor air sample for formaldehyde and measured indoor temperature and relative humidity. They also administered a short questionnaire to adult residents about occupant demographics and trailer characteristics, and they conducted a walk-through survey of the exterior and interior of sampled units. The geometric mean level of formaldehyde in sampled trailers was 77 ppb (range: 3–590 ppb). The geometric mean formaldehyde level was 81 ppb for travel trailers (95% CI: 72–92), 44 ppb for park models (95% CI: 38–53), and 57 ppb for manufactured homes (95% CI: 49–65). Formaldehyde levels varied by trailer type, but all types tested had at least one sample result with levels≥ 100 ppb, the level at which health effects have been described in sensitive persons.[5]

CDC also worked with Lawrence Berkeley National Laboratory (LBNL) under an Interagency Agreement to try to determine the specific sources of formaldehyde in the travel trailers. Air samples were taken from four different makes and models of previously occupied travel trailers. These samples were analyzed for formaldehyde, VOCs (a screening of several dozen different compounds) and acetic acid. Samples of the trailer building materials were then removed from the trailers and shipped to LBNL's facility, where the samples were placed in chambers to determine the material's emission rates for formaldehyde, VOCs, and acetic acid. In addition to formaldehyde, acetic acid, phenol, and 2,2,4-trimethyl-1,3-pentanediol di-isobutyrate (TMPD-DIB) were found in the air at concentrations higher than typically seen from comparative housing in the United States. While the emission rates from the materials were generally lower than the U.S. Department of Housing and Urban Development (HUD) Standard[6] for manufactured housing (not applicable to travel trailers), the high measures of formaldehyde concentrations were attributed to the high loading of formaldehyde-emitting material combined with the low air exchange rate in the trailers.

Finally, as related to this current project, CDC was also asked to assess potential mitigation strategies to control formaldehyde concentrations in trailers. CDC established an Interagency Agreement with NASA to jointly conduct this mitigation research. In the project reported here, 17 never-occupied travel trailers (15 for testing, 2 as dummy trailers) provided a controlled test environment for evaluating the effectiveness of a variety of air cleaning or ventilation-related devices for reducing the formaldehyde concentrations in the indoor environment. This project was designed to provide initial information on each mitigation device's ability to reduce indoor formaldehyde levels.

The seventeen trailers selected for this investigation were Cavalier models manufactured by Gulfstream Coach to FEMA's specifications specifically for use following Hurricanes Katrina and Rita. The trailers were the same make and model, and they were manufactured on the same day (April 5, 2006), in the same plant (VIN plant ID #1, location unknown). CDC personnel inspected each trailer to ensure it was free of obvious water leaks and water damage and that it was in good condition (e.g., walls not bowing, no exterior or interior material damage). FEMA transported the trailers from the FEMA storage lot in Selma, Alabama to the Stennis Space Center in Mississippi for electrical hookup and testing.

4) TECHNOLOGY SELECTION APPROACH

Two different strategies for mitigating formaldehyde in travel trailers have been proposed by various individuals and groups: treatments and add-on devices. Treatments of the trailers can generally be thought of as one-time events, such as the application of a compound in a trailer to reduce or eliminate formaldehyde generation. These applications generally involve hazardous compounds and would need to be carried out in a carefully controlled manner. While they have not been rejected as ineffective, treatments were not included in this investigation due to the differences in mitigation approaches (i.e., treatment of the building material rather than treatment of the air).

Add-on devices, the focus of this research, included air cleaners and ventilation units. To be included in this evaluation, the mitigation approach needed to incorporate some type of technology that appeared to be capable of removing formaldehyde from the air. Some air cleaning units were particulate filtering units only; these units were excluded from the evaluation. Technologies specifically claiming to release ozone to remove air contaminants were eliminated from consideration in this evaluation because of health hazards associated with ozone exposures.[7] Beyond these exclusions, all other technologies were considered for the evaluation.

A review of the reaction kinetics between formaldehyde and ozone indicated the reaction is relatively slow. To drive this reaction forward, high concentrations of ozone would be required to sufficiently reduce the formaldehyde concentrations. These high ozone concentrations would present a potential respiratory hazard to the residents, and they could represent the trading of one hazard (formaldehyde) for a different one (ozone). In addition, ozone is highly reactive, with the potential of reacting with other

11

compounds in the trailer environment. Because of the complex nature of the trailer environment, ozone reaction products may also represent a hazard to the residents. All units, with the exception of the ventilation-based devices, were evaluated for ozone generation before being included in the evaluation. This evaluation consisted of operating the unit in a laboratory, measuring the ozone concentration of the air at the outlet of the device with a UV-based ozone monitor, and comparing that measurement with a measurement of the laboratory background concentration. Devices that had a significantly higher ozone concentration at the outlet (more than double the laboratory concentration, and in no case was the output concentration more than 10.5ppb) were excluded from the evaluation. A detailed description of the ozone testing and the results are given in Appendix A.

In addition to a test of every unit for ozone, several units were evaluated for ultraviolet (UV) light emissions. The photocatalytic oxidation units use UV light as a part of the oxidation process. Those photocatalytic oxidation units in which the UV light source was visibly exposed were tested for their emissions. One of these units was excluded from the trailer evaluation due to high UV light emissions. A detailed description of the UV light emission testing and the results are given in Appendix A.

5) MITIGATION TECHNOLOGIES

Four different technology categories were evaluated: ventilation, oxidation, diffusion/adsorption, and ionization. A general description of each technology category is provided in the subsections that follow. Table 1 provides information regarding each of the specific devices that were tested. Technologies considered for this investigation were either identified through a literature search, or they were brought to the researchers' attention by project partners or by representatives of the companies producing or selling a device.

a. Ventilation

Ventilation involves removing indoor air, which removes indoor air contaminants, and bringing in outside air, thus diluting the concentration of contaminants in the trailer. The challenge with ventilation is that, depending on the weather, bringing in large volumes of unconditioned air could easily overburden the heating and cooling systems installed in these trailers. This is particularly critical in the hot, humid summer months. If ventilation results in high indoor temperature and humidity, emission rates of formaldehyde from the building products could increase and, depending on the ventilation rate, may result in higher formaldehyde concentrations. To overcome this problem, one evaluated ventilating unit incorporated energy recovery capabilities to precondition incoming air, thereby increasing the ventilation rate while helping to maintain the indoor trailer environment at an acceptable temperature and humidity.

Another type of ventilation control is a powered roof vent. Most of the travel trailers are built with at least one powered roof vent in the bathroom, and occasionally one in the kitchen. One vendor markets an add-on device that provides a three-speed fan built into an enclosure that covers the existing roof vent. This enclosure design allows the fan to exhaust air from the trailer while protecting the interior from rain; it is not amenable to the side-vented kitchen exhaust present on many travel trailers. The level of protection from the elements is one of the major advantages of this add-on device over the trailer manufacturer-installed vents. This new vent was installed over the existing roof vent. The fan was rated at 500, 680, and 982 Cubic feet per Minute (CFM) for each of the fan speeds low, medium, and high, respectively, and was operated at its maximum speed. A trailer air exchange rate test (See the "Determination of Air Exchange Rates" section later in this document) was conducted both with and without the fan running to determine the actual exhaust flow rate.[8]

Another ventilation solution involved the replacement of the manufacturer-installed air conditioning system with a system that provided a small amount of outside air to the trailer. This replacement system functioned much like the originally installed system; however, a small vent was provided in the side of the return air plenum. A small deflector was installed over the vent to prevent the entry of water into the plenum Operation of the air conditioner's fan placed the return air plenum under negative pressure. This drew outside air into the plenum, which was then distributed throughout the trailer. The exact volume of outside air drawn into the plenum was not specified by the manufacturer; rather, it was determined through the air exchange rate test run both with and without the vent sealed.

b. Oxidation

Four different oxidation solutions were evaluated: photocatalytic oxidation, potassium permanganate, and two filter treatments. Photocatalytic oxidation (PCO) utilizes ultraviolet or near-ultraviolet wavelength (< 385 nm) radiation to promote electrons from the valence band into the conduction band of a titanium dioxide semiconductor. Reactions with molecular oxygen or hydroxyl radicals destroy volatile organic compounds, and super-oxide ions form after the initial production of highly reactive electron-hole pairs. While PCO can completely oxidize VOCs, a "complete" conversion is difficult to document because a carbon mass balance is limited by the analytical methods used to quantify possible intermediate products. Intermediate products from the oxidation of organic compounds are likely to include aldehydes, ketones, esters, and acids.[9]

Potassium permanganate is an oxidizer that will react with aldehydes to form carboxylic acids. In the case of formaldehyde, formic acid is formed as a by-product. In the device tested in the FEMA-owned trailers, alumina was impregnated with potassium permanganate, and this sorbent was placed inside a HEPA filter used in an off-the-shelf portable air cleaner.

Two additional oxidation control methods were assessed in this investigation. In both cases, filter media were treated with proprietary mixtures that reportedly react with formaldehyde in the air. The first contained a mixture of food-grade compounds that was applied to filter media; this media was installed into the filter holder of the trailer's air conditioning system. The second mixture contained several hydrazine-related

15

compounds; the mixture was applied to the HEPA filter of a portable room air cleaner. At this time, no additional information on the composition of these two filter treatment compounds is available.

c. Diffusion/Adsorption

A single product relying on passive diffusion/adsorption was assessed. This product was a zeolite material sealed in a Tyvek® pouch. The material reportedly adsorbs formaldehyde as well as a wide variety of other compounds. Because air is not actively moved across the material, contaminants from within the trailer would have to diffuse into the packets to be captured. Each packet contained approximately 400 grams of the zeolite material; according to the manufacturer, a packet could treat approximately 100 ft^2. Three packets were used in the test trailer, as recommended by the manufacturer. The packets were not replaced during the test. This product is inexpensive (relative to the other tested devices) and easily replaceable.

d. Ionization

The ionization technologies evaluated here included: reactive oxygen species, cold plasma, bipolar ionization, and quadruple ion technology. While the method for generating ions varied between the different technologies, in general, most generated oxygen-related ions. Ozone generation appeared to be a potential problem with many of the ionization technologies.

e. Reactive Oxygen Species

Reactive Oxygen Species is a technology by which a limited amount of the oxygen in a room is converted to one of several species, such as superoxide, hydrogen peroxide, and hydroxyl radical.[10] These molecules then oxidize organic compounds similar to the other oxidation-based devices. Only one device identified uses Reactive Oxygen Species, and it was not clear from the company literature how it was generating these compounds.[11]

f. Cold Plasma

With cold plasma, ultraviolet (UV) light at 100–280 nm generates cold gas plasma, in addition to breaking bonds in many organic compounds. One source reported generating atomic oxygen, molecular singlet oxygen, and activated oxygen species.[12] Another source specifically mentioned the use of cold plasma for the production of ozone.[13] A single manufacturer of this type of device provided a unit for evaluation.[14]

g. Bipolar Ionization

With bipolar ionization, air is drawn past an ionization tube containing two electrodes. Both positive and negative ions are generated, and these ions react with oxygen, which then reacts with a variety of organic compounds. One source specifically mentioned the production of ozone with this technology.[15] A single manufacturer of this type of device provided a unit for evaluation.[16]

h. Quadruple Ion Technology

Quadruple ion technology uses moisture in the air, as well as the air itself, to generate four reactive compounds: hydrogen peroxide (H_2O_2), hydroxyl radical (HO), super oxide ion (O_2^-), and ozonide ion (O_3^-). These four compounds react with various volatile organic compounds. The single manufacturer of the device using quadruple ion technology claimed there is little ozone generated by the technology.[17]

Sixteen different devices were selected for evaluation, as shown in Table 1. Photographs of these units as installed in the travel trailers are provided in Appendix B.

Table 1. Mitigation devices considered for selection in the evaluation. Gray shaded devices were not evaluated in the test trailers due to high ozone output. Pink shaded devices were not evaluated in the test trailers due to high UV light output.

Trailer – Device	Company	Technology	Website
1–Formal X	So-Brite Chemicals International, Inc.	Treated Filter	http://www.dsr5.com/contact.htm
2–Forever Fresh	Worldwide Sales, Inc.	Passive diffusion/ adsorption	http://www.foreverfresh.us/index.htm
3–Prototype	Safehome	Potassium Permanganate	https://www.safehomefilters.com/
5–HEPAiRx	Air Innovations	Ventilation	http://www.airinnovations.com/
6–AiroCide	KES	Photocatalytic Oxidation	http://www.kesscience.com/
7–S900	Airsopure	Photocatalytic Oxidation	http://www.asopure.com/en/products/residential.html
7–Prototype	ANGUS Chemical	Treated Filter	http://www.dow.com/angus/
8–Eraldehyde	MicroSweep Corp	Treated Filter	http://www.microsweep.com/
9–MaxxAir Turbo/ Maxx™ - 3550	Maxxair Vent Co.	Ventilation	http://www.maxxair.com/Products/Turbo-Maxx.aspx
10–Prototype	Fluid Lines	Photocatalytic Oxidation	
11–Prototype	PURETi	Photocatalytic Oxidation	http://www.pureti.com/home.html
11–Prototype	Texas A&M University	Photocatalytic Oxidation	
12–Prototype	Nanocepts	Photocatalytic Oxidation	http://www.nanocepts.com/
13–Prototype	Aria Acqua	Photocatalytic Oxidation	
14–AirOcare	AirOcare	Reactive Oxygen Species	http://www.airocare.com/
15–Coleman-Mach Air Conditioner	Airxcel, Inc	Ventilation	http://www.rvcomfort.com/rvp/products/rooftop/rooftop.php
Nanobreeze	NanoTwin Technologies	Photocatalytic Oxidation	http://nanotwin.com/
Prototype	ActiveTek	ActivePure Technology (H_2O_2)	http://www.activtek.net/ProductDetail/tabid/154/Default.aspx?Product=US40532
AF1000	Air Fantastic	Quadruple Ion Technology	http://www.airfantastic.com/
Prototype	AERISA	Cold Plasma	http://www.aerisa.com/
AtmosAir T-400	Clean Air Group	Bipolar Ionization	http://www.atmosair.com/

19

6) STUDY DESIGN

This evaluation initially involved the assessment of 14 different mitigation solutions, as described in the previous section. As the sampling data results were received, it became clear that three of the tested devices were ineffective. In two cases, these ineffective devices were replaced with two devices that were not included in the original 14 units tested. While the results for the two additional devices are limited, they provide some indication of their performance. The final list of evaluated units was dependent upon the initial assessment of ozone and UV light emission from each device. Each solution was set up in one trailer and continuously operated throughout the test period (with the exception of the three mentioned ineffective devices and two replacements).

The test trailers were placed on a crushed limestone site side-by-side approximately 8 feet apart and with the same orientation to the sun. Fifteen travel trailers were sampled in this evaluation; fourteen trailers contained a mitigation technology and one trailer served as a control. The remaining two trailers were not involved in sampling and were placed at either end of the row of trailers to ensure that all trailers experienced similar solar loading. Each test trailer was provided with electrical power to run the air conditioning system, portable heaters, mitigation devices, and necessary sampling equipment. The trailer volume was approximately 40 m^3 (1400 ft^3). Assignment of the control devices to the different trailers was random.

The inside of the test trailers had the same configuration and furnishings. The bedroom door was completely opened. The door to the bathroom was fixed at the half-opened position by a doorstop. All cabinets and drawers throughout the trailer were partially opened. All window treatments (curtains, blinds, etc.) were completely opened. Bathroom vents were closed (except for the ventilation technology that used a fan in the bathroom vent). The air conditioning fan was set to operate continuously to promote mixing within the trailer. The air conditioning system's thermostat was set to approximately 72°F. As weather conditions would likely result in ambient temperature well below 72°F, all trailers were provided with a small space heater set to approximately 65°F. No appliances were operated, nor were water or sewer lines connected. Water was added to each sink, tub drain, and toilet to ensure that there were no dry plumbing traps. Water levels were checked weekly and additional water added as necessary.

7) METHODOLOGY

The data collect in this evaluation included air samples for aldehydes, including formaldehyde, VOCs, acetic acid, and TMPD-DIB. The complete list of compounds and the associated methods are given in Table 2. Indoor and outdoor temperature and humidity measurements were made over the entire term of the project. Ambient wind speed and direction were also collected. In addition, air exchange rates were measured during two different periods to determine air exchange rates for each trailer and the air exchange rates of trailers with the ventilation-based solutions operating. The methods and procedures for collecting these data are provided later in this report.

a. Air Sampling—Analytical Methods

Aldehydes, including formaldehyde, were sampled and analyzed via EPA Method TO-11A.[18] Initially, these samples were also analyzed for twelve different aldehydes (see list in Table 2). However, initial sample results showed detectable concentrations only for formaldehyde and acetaldehyde. Beginning on February 9, 2009, sample analysis was scaled back to formaldehyde and acetaldehyde only, with the full aldehyde screening occurring once every other week. Sampling occurred for 1 hour, with a flow rate of approximately 500 milliliters per minute (ml/min). The limit of quantitation (LOQ) was 0.2 µg/sample, resulting in a minimum quantifiable concentration of 6 ppb with a 30-liter air sample volume.

Table 2. List of compounds to be quantified, by analytical method.

Aldehydes, EPA Method TO-11A		VOCs EPA Method TO-17		
formaldehyde	acetaldehyde	propene	dichlorodi-fluoromethane	chloromethane
propion-aldehyde	crotonaldehyde	Freon 114	vinyl chloride	1,3-butadiene
n-butyl-aldehyde	benzaldehyde	bromo-methane	chloroethane	ethanol
Isovaler-aldehyde	valeraldehyde	isopropyl alcohol	Freon 11	cis-1,2-dichloroethane
o-tolualdehyde	m,p-tolu-aldehyde	carbon disulfide	Freon 113	acetone
hexaldehyde	2,5-dimethyl-benzaldehyde	methylene chloride	trans-1,2-dichloro-ethane	1,1-dichloroethane
		methyl t-butyl ether	vinyl acetate	1,1-dichloroethene
TMPD-DIB, OSHA Method PV2002		2-butanone	ethyl acetate	hexane
2,2,4-trimethyl-1,3-pentanediol di-isobutyrate (TMPD-DIB)		chloroform	1,1,1-trichloro-ethane	carbon tetrachloride
		benzene	tetrahydrofuran	1,2-dichloro-ethane
VOCs EPA Method TO-17 Tentatively Identified		cyclohexane	trichloroethene	heptane
hexanal	unknown amine	1,2-dichloro-propane	bromodichloro-methane	cis-1,3-di-chloro-propene
α-pinene	phenol	4-metyl-2-pentanone	toluene	trans-1,3-dichloropropene
octanal	nonanal	1,1,2-tri-chloroethane	tetrachloro-ethene	2-hexanone
decanal	C13 hydrocarbon	dibromochloro-methane	1,2-dibromo-methane	chlorobenzene
tetradecane	acetic acid	ethylbenzene	M,p-xylene	o-xylene
propanoic acid	butane	styrene	bromoform	1,1,2,2-tetra-chlorethane
2-methyl-butane	2-hexenal	benzyl chloride	4-ethyl toluene	1,3,5-trimethyl-benzene
tridecane	propane	1,2,4-tri-methylbenzene	1,3-dichloro-benzene	1,4-dichloro-benzene
pentane	unknown acid ester	1,2-dichloro-benzene	1,2,4-trichloro-benzene	Hexachloro-butadiene
		Acetic Acid, NIOSH Method 1603		
		acetic acid		

Volatile Organic Compounds were collected and analyzed by EPA method TO-17.[19] One-hour samples were collected at an approximate air flow rate of 200 ml/min (±5%). The method specifies a minimum detection limit of 25 ng/sample. A 12-liter air sample volume provided a minimum quantifiable concentration of 2.1 ppb.

TMPD-DIB was sampled and analyzed by OSHA method PV2002.[20] One-hour samples were collected at an approximate air flow rate of 200 ml/min (±5%). This sampling rate is higher than method specifications; however, communication with OSHA indicated 200 ml/min is an acceptable maximum flow rate.[21] This sample volume will yield a minimum reliable quantitation concentration of approximately 70 ppb. Initial sample results showed no detectable concentrations of TMPD-DIB in any of the samples. Therefore, no samples were collected for TMPD after January 26, 2009.

Acetic acid was sampled and analyzed by modified National Institute for Occupational Safety and Health (NIOSH) method 1603.[21, 22] Lower detection limits, 2 µg/sample, were achieved by using ion chromatography with a conductivity detector, rather than high-pressure liquid chromatography with an ultraviolet detector, as specified in the method. One-hour samples were collected at an approximate air flow rate of 400 ml/min (±5%). This yielded a minimum quantifiable concentration of 34 ppb.

b. Air Sampling—Field Procedures

Each trailer's kitchen table window was slightly modified to accommodate air sampling equipment. A panel of polycarbonate was cut to fit on the outside of the window. Three holes, two for sample tube insertion and one to allow the original window to open, were drilled into the plastic. The panel was sealed with aluminum tape. When sampling was not occurring, the three holes were sealed. A small shelf was installed below the window to hold the sampling pumps.

The sampling media were placed on one end of 4-ft long, ¼ in ID stainless steel tubing. The other end of the stainless steel tubing was connected to the inlet of the appropriately calibrated sampling pump via Tygon tubing. The sampling tubes with the sampling media connected were inserted into the trailer interior through pre-drilled holes in the plastic window panel so that the sample media were suspended in the isle between the kitchen table and cabinets, at the approximate longitudinal centerline of the trailers and at the approximate mid-point between the floor and ceiling. The holes where the stainless steel tubes were inserted through the window panel were sealed with aluminum foil. A photograph of the air sampling equipment setup is given in Figure 1.

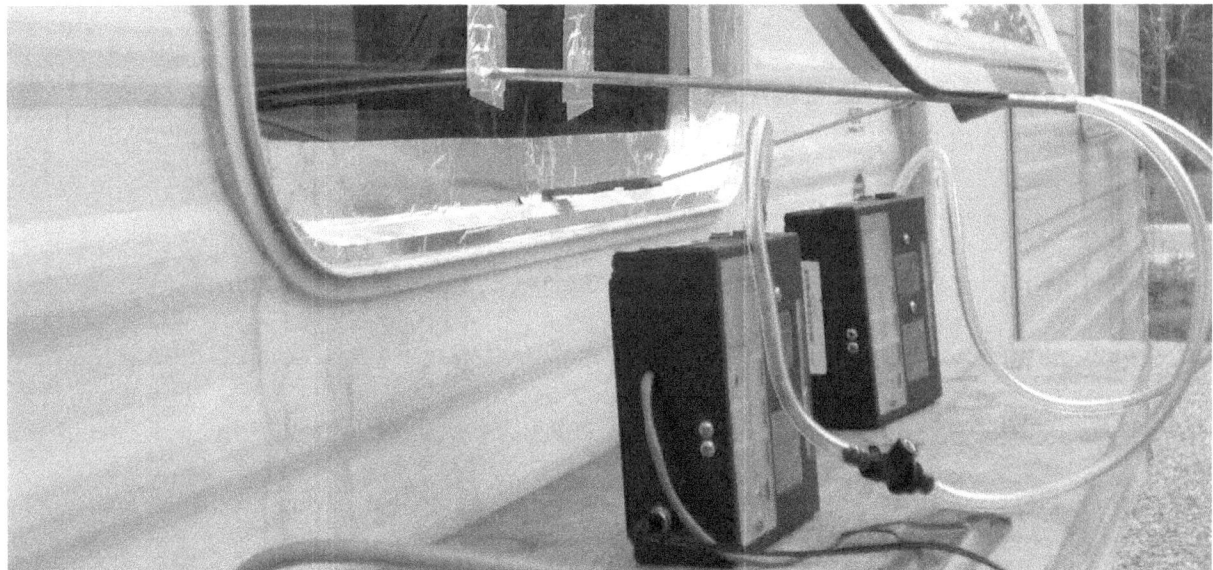

Figure 1. Air sampling equipment setup outside of travel trailer.

Initially, the aldehyde sampling pumps were configured to operate on AC power, rather than battery power, for improved pump reliability. AC power was available through receptacles located on the outside of the trailers. However, the cycling of the trailers'

25

air conditioning systems appeared to result in voltage drops that caused the pumps to fault. Beginning on March 2, 2009, the aldehyde pumps were operated on battery power. Pre- and post- pump calibration was performed where the trailers were staged. Appendix C contains specific quality assurance and quality control information for sample collection, storage, and shipment. Sampling data (pump and calibrator serial numbers, start/stop times, calibration flow rates, sample numbers, etc.) were entered into sample data sheets shown in Appendix D. Chain of custody was maintained. Samples were analyzed by an American Board of Industrial Hygiene-accredited laboratory (DataChem) with documented proficiency in formaldehyde analysis. Documented proficiency was shown by participation in the workplace analysis scheme for proficiency (WASP) program.

In addition to the samples collected inside the trailers, a similar set of ambient samples was collected to document the environmental conditions. These samples were collected near the base of the meteorological station approximately five feet above the ground.

Table 3 shows the sampling schedule. The sampling schedule was developed to maximize samples on the basis of available resources. Samples were collected relatively simultaneously; all pumps were started within an hour of each other in the early afternoon. The pump start-up order was randomly assigned for each sampling day.

Baseline samples (no mitigation units operational) were collected daily for two one-week periods prior to starting the different mitigation devices. At the end of Week 14, the mitigation devices were shut off and/or removed from the trailers. The trailers were allowed to sit undisturbed for two weeks (Weeks 15 and 16) with heaters and air conditioners operating; then the final two weeks of sampling (Weeks 17 and 18) were conducted as a second set of baseline samples. Sampling results from the first week of baseline sampling (Week 0) were received prior to the initiation of the mitigation devices. This schedule allowed for modifications to the original sampling design as necessary. For example, the flow rate for the acetic acid sampling was reduced from 800 ml/min to 400 ml/min to avoid potential breakthrough onto the second (back) half of the sample media.

Samples for aldehydes, including formaldehyde, were collected on each sampling day; one of the other three compounds/compound categories was usually sampled at the same time as the formaldehyde sample on a rotating basis. On the basis of sampling results obtained, TMPD-DIB sampling was discontinued after January 26, 2009; on the days when TMPD-DIB would have been sampled, only aldehyde sampling occurred. In addition, aldehyde analysis was scaled back twice on the basis of ongoing review of air sample results. Initially, aldehyde samples were analyzed for all twelve aldehydes listed in Table 2. Since the only detected compounds were formaldehyde and acetaldehyde, on February 2, 2009, the analysis was limited to only these two compounds on each sampling day, except for full twelve-compound analyses once every other week. After March 12, 2009, all aldehyde sampling analyses were limited to formaldehyde and acetaldehyde.

Table 3. Sampling Schedule

	Week	Sun	Mon	Tue	Wed	Thu	Fri	Sat
Week 0 (Baseline)	12/14/08	Dec 15	16	17 V A	18 T F-Full	19 A F-Full	20 V T	21
Week 1 (Baseline)	01/11/09	Jan 11	12	13 A F-Full	14 T F-Full	15 A F-Full	16 V F-Full	17 V F-Full
Week 2 (Reactors Installed)	01/18/09	18 F-Full	19 V F-Full	20 F-Full A	21 T F-Full	22 F-Full	23 A F-Full	14 T F-Full
Week 3	01/25/09	25 F-Full	26 T F-Full	27	28 V F-Full	29	30 A F-Full	31
Week 4	02/01/09	Feb 1	2 V F-Full	3	4 A F	5	6 F T	7
Week 5	02/08/09	8	9 A F	10	11	12 F-Full	13	14
Week 6	02/15/09	15	16	17 A F	18	19	20 V F	21
Week 7	02/22/09	22	23 A F	24	25	26 F-Full	27	28
Week 8	03/01/09	Mar 1	2 A F	3	4	5 V F	6	7
Week 9	03/08/09	8	9 A F	10	11	12 F-Full	13	14
Week 10	03/15/09	15	16 A F	17	18	19 V F	20	21
Week 11	03/22/09	22	23 A F	24	25	26 F	27	28
Week 12	03/29/09	29	30 A F	31	Apr 1	2 V F	3	4
Week 13	04/05/09	5	6 A F	7	8	9 F	10	11
Week 14	04/12/09	12	13 A F	14	15	16 V F	17	18
Week 15 (No sampling)	04/19/09	19	20	21	22	23	24	25
Week 16 (No sampling)	04/26/09	26	27	28	29	30	May 1	2
Week 17 (Baseline)	05/03/09	3	4 A F	5	6 V F	7	8 A F	9
Week 18 (Baseline)	05/10/09	10	11 A F	12	13 V F	14	15 A F	16

A=acetic acid   F=formaldehyde and acetaldehyde only   F-Full=Full aldehyde scan   T=TMPD-DIB   V=VOCs

c. Temperature and Relative Humidity

Trailer temperature and relative humidity measurements were made near the center of each THU's primary living room using HOBO brand temperature and relative humidity logging monitors (Onset Computer Corporation, Bourne, Massachusetts). The HOBOs were placed on the kitchen countertop, near the edge of the counter closest to the kitchen table. They were placed out of direct sunlight. The HOBOs were set to log data continuously at 5-minute intervals, and were downloaded and reprogrammed every two to three weeks over the course of the evaluation.

A meteorological station collected outdoor environmental condition data, including air temperature, relative humidity, barometric pressure, wind speed, wind direction, and solar irradiance. The station consisted of a temperature/humidity probe (Campbell Scientific HMP50 Temperature/Humidity Probe), an anemometer (R.M. Young 05305 Anemometer), a barometer (Campbell Scientific CS105 Barometric Pressure Sensor), and a pyranometer (Eppley PSP Precision Spectral Pyranometer). The station was mounted on a 2-meter tripod support and positioned near the center of the row of 17 trailers; it was offset approximately 8 meters from the row. Measurements were recorded at one-minute intervals and automatically stored on a data logger. The meteorological station data logger was downloaded at similar frequencies and times as the HOBO temperature and humidity monitors.

d. Determination of Air Exchange Rates

The air exchange rates for each trailer were measured two or three times on different days, both before air sampling began and after all air sampling was completed. The concentration decay test method and regression method in the ASTM Standard Test Method for Determining Air Change in a Single Zone by Means of a Tracer Gas Dilution (ASTM E 741-00 [Reapproved 2006]) was used, utilizing carbon dioxide (CO_2).[23] For any trailer testing a ventilation solution, the air exchange rate was determined both with and without the ventilation unit running. Pure CO_2 was released as a burst into the return of the air-conditioning system and allowed to mix for 30 minutes. The decay was monitored for a minimum of 1 hour. Throughout the entire test period, the trailer's air conditioner was set at 72°F to match the conditions during the sampling periods. The trailer was not entered during the decay period. During both the mixing and the decay periods, carbon dioxide levels were measured with a Q-Trak indoor air quality monitor (TSI Incorporated, Shoreview, Minnesota). A Q-Trak was also set up to measure the outdoor CO_2 concentration at the meteorological station location. The Q-Trak's probe was placed on the kitchen table near the edge closest to the longitudinal center line of the trailer. The instrument display was positioned so that the concentration of CO_2 could be read through the window of the trailer. The Q-Trak was configured to log data at 30-second intervals and was operated and calibrated according to the manufacturer's directions. The order of testing was determined by random assignment of numbers to each trailer, including both the ventilation-on and ventilation-off configurations. The air exchange rate was determined by calculating the slope of the linear portion of the plot of the natural logarithm of the difference of the indoor and ambient CO_2 concentrations versus time. This slope was determined by running a linear regression on a one-hour segment of the data once the concentration in the trailer had stabilized, where the natural logarithm concentration versus time plot was linear.

8) DATA ANALYSIS and RESULTS

a. Trailer Air Exchange Data

As described in the **METHODOLOGY** section of this report, trailer air exchange rates were measured both before sampling began and after sampling was completed. The air exchange rate was determined from the slope of the best fit line (as determined from a linear regression) for the plot of the natural logarithm of the difference between the in-trailer and ambient CO_2 concentrations versus time. Table 4 shows the calculated trailer air exchange rates for the measurements made before sampling began. Each trailer and ventilation configuration was measured at least twice, with four trailers measured a third time. Table 4 also provides the means and standard deviations of these measurements. The coefficient of determination (R^2) values for the linear regressions to determine the pre-sampling air exchange rates were between 0.9919 and 0.9999. Table 5 provides similar results for the post-sampling measurements of air exchange rates. The R^2 values for the linear regressions to determine the post-sampling air exchange rates were between 0.9479 and 0.9999. This narrow range indicates that individual air exchange rates remained constant throughout the air exchange test.

Table 4. Pre-sampling measured trailer ventilation rates, in air changes per hour (ACH), with means and standard deviations.

Trailer/ Technology	Ventilation	Test 1 Date/ Time	Test 1 Result	Test 2 Date/ Time	Test 2 Result	Test 3 Date/ Time	Test 3 Result	Mean	STD
1 Remov	No	11/19/08 15:04	0.898	11/21/08 8:32	1.02			0.961	0.0891
2 Forever Fresh	No	11/19/08 15:03	0.630	11/20/08 7:50	0.696			0.663	0.0464
3 Safehome	No	11/19/08 15:00	0.948	11/21/08 8:35	0.982			0.965	0.0240
4 Control	No	11/19/08 14:56	0.841	11/20/08 9:34	0.817			0.829	0.0168
5 HEPAir X	No	11/19/08 14:55	0.757	11/21/08 8:37	0.842			0.800	0.0596
	Yes	11/20/08 10:59	1.34	11/20/08 14:11	3.02			2.18	1.19
6 KES	No	11/19/08 13:18	0.956	11/20/08 9:37	0.881	11/20/08 15:49	1.09	0.976	0.106
7 AirsoPure /ANGUS Chem	No	11/19/08 13:16	0.796	11/20/08 11:05	0.811			0.804	0.0110
8 Eralde-hyde	No	11/19/08 13:13	0.722	11/20/08 12:32	0.805			0.764	0.0590
9 MaxxAir	No	11/19/08 13:06	0.930	11/21/08 8:39	0.854			0.892	0.0540
	Yes	11/20/08 11:09	13.9	11/20/08 14:14	15.3			14.6	1.01
10 Fluid Lines	No	11/19/08 13:04	0.753	11/20/08 12:39	0.715	11/20/08 15:52	0.767	0.745	0.0271
11 Texas A&M/ Pureti	No	11/19/08 11:41	0.778	11/20/08 12:43	0.755			0.767	0.0166
12 Nano-cepts	No	11/19/08 11:39	0.776	11/20/08 12:46	0.741	11/20/08 15:54	0.752	0.757	0.0177
13 Aria Acqua	No	11/19/08 11:36	0.918	11/20/08 14:17	0.929			0.923	0.00816
14 AiroCare	No	11/19/08 11:31	1.05	11/20/08 9:40	0.949	11/20/08 15:57	1.00	1.00	0.0511
15 Airxcel	No	11/19/08 11:27	0.507	11/21/08 8:43	0.515			0.511	0.00585
	Yes	11/20/08 11:13	1.05	11/20/08 14:22	1.01			1.03	0.0340

Table 5. Post-sampling measured trailer ventilation rates, in air changes per hour (ACH), with means and standard deviations.

Trailer/Technology	Ventilation	Test 1 Date/Time	Test 1 Result	Test 2 Date/Time	Test 2 Result	Test 3 Date/Time	Test 3 Result	Mean	STD
1 Remov	No	5/19/09 10:53	0.838	5/20/09 8:04	0.795	5/21/09 13:43	0.800	0.811	0.0240
2 Forever Fresh	No	5/19/09 8:37	0.723	5/20/09 10:00	0.758	5/21/09 14:49	0.753	0.745	0.0188
3 Safehome	No	5/19/09 10:50	1.04	5/20/09 12:36	1.04	5/21/09 10:02	0.917	1.00	0.0719
4 Control	No	5/19/09 12:58	0.886	5/20/09 14:38	0.815	5/21/09 10:07	0.839	0.847	0.0356
5 HEPAir X	No	5/19/09 14:55	0.839	5/20/09 12:45	0.888	5/21/09 8:01	0.749	0.825	0.0704
	Yes	Not measured							
6 KES	No	5/19/09 14:52	0.904	5/20/09 9:57	0.872	5/21/09 8:09	0.851	0.876	0.0266
7 AirsoPure /ANGUS Chem	No	5/19/09 14:57	0.914	5/20/09 8:14	0.832	5/21/09 11:52	0.747	0.831	0.0835
8 Eraldehyde	No	5/19/09 14:59	0.808	5/20/09 12:42	0.871	5/21/09 13:39	0.717	0.802	0.0786
9 MaxxAir	No	5/19/09 13:01	0.888	5/20/09 12:39	0.949	5/21/09 13:37	0.872	0.903	0.0405
	Yes	5/19/09 16:44	12.6	5/20/09 8:01	12.9	5/20/09 14:45	11.7	12.4	0.608
10 Fluid Lines	No	5/19/09 8:31	0.799	5/19/09 16:52	0.717	5/21/09 9:58	0.745	0.754	0.0419
11 Texas A&M/ Pureti	No	5/19/09 8:29	0.732	5/20/09 10:04	0.723	5/21/09 11:54	0.665	0.707	0.0365
12 Nanocepts	No	5/19/09 8:34	0.817	5/19/09 16:46	0.739	5/21/09 11:50	0.690	0.749	0.0638
13 Aria Acqua	No	5/19/09 10:56	0.977	5/20/09 10:07	0.908	5/21/09 8:05	0.909	0.931	0.0400
14 AirOcare	No	5/19/09 12:56	0.958	5/20/09 8:09	0.873	5/21/09 11:57	0.863	0.898	0.0524
15 Airxcel	No	5/19/09 10:46	0.610	5/19/09 16:49	0.530	5/21/09 10:11	0.513	0.551	0.0515
	Yes	5/19/09 13:04	1.09	5/20/09 14:41	1.04	5/21/09 7:59	1.17	1.10	0.0635

b. Temperature and Relative Humidity Data

Temperature and relative humidity plots for the trailers and ambient conditions are shown in Appendix E. Each plot shows the temperature or relative humidity for each trailer and the ambient measurement over a given period of time. Other atmospheric data, including solar irradiance, wind speed and direction, and barometric pressure, were collected by the meteorological station; these data have not been fully assessed and may be further evaluated in the future.

c. Air Sampling Data

Quality assurance/quality control measures in sample collection, shipment, and laboratory analysis were followed. Laboratory quality assurance parameters (e.g., percent recovery of spike samples) were within the acceptable analytical method limits.

The sample results received from the contract laboratory were reported as a mass of analyte per sample. For all the sampling methods, concentrations were calculated by use of equation 1,

$$C = 24450 \times \frac{m}{V \times MW} \qquad (1)$$

Where: C = concentration (ppb),

m = mass of analyte (μg),

V = sample volume (l), and

MW = molecular weight of analyte.

The sample volume was determined by calculating the average of the pre- and post-calibration pump flow rates and multiplying by the sample duration. The calculated sample concentrations for aldehydes (including formaldehyde), acetic acid, and TMPD-DIB, along with the sample dates, trailer numbers, sample durations, sample volumes, and sample mass, are given in Appendix F. Appendix G provides similar data for those VOC compounds that were detected or tentatively identified.

Air samples for TMPD-DIB were collected as outlined in Table 3; all samples, both baseline and evaluation samples, were non-detected for TMPD-DIB. Formaldehyde was detected in every trailer sample. The range of mean values was 108–310 ppb in the pre-evaluation baseline samples; 48–432 ppb in the evaluation samples; and 154–418 ppb in the post-evaluation baseline samples. Acetaldehyde was not detected in the pre-evaluation baseline samples. Its concentration ranged from 3.7–10.6 ppb in the evaluation samples and from 3.5–6.3 ppb in the post-evaluation baseline samples. Acetic acid values ranged from 103–316 ppb in the pre-evaluation baseline samples; from 66–220 ppb in the evaluation samples; and from 60–124 ppb in the post-evaluation baseline samples. Summary data for formaldehyde and acetaldehyde, the only aldehydes detected, as well as acetic acid results are given in Table 6.

Table 6. Summary concentration data (ppb) for formaldehyde, acetaldehyde, and acetic acid samples.

	Pre-evaluation Baseline Samples											
Trailer No	Formaldehyde				Acetaldehyde				Acetic Acid			
	Mean	n	Min	Max	Mean	n+	Min	Max	Mean	n	Min	Max
1	310	7	150	678	*	*	*	*	254	4	172	450
2	117	7	53	274	*	*	*	*	183	4	127	324
3	125	7	54	267	*	*	*	*	119	4	78	210
4	123	7	62	264	*	*	*	*	185	4	153	266
5	170	7	101	377	*	*	*	*	168	4	143	185
6	170	7	83	373	*	*	*	*	126	4	104	165
7	138	7	51	311	*	*	*	*	116	4	102	141
8	257	7	119	542	*	*	*	*	216	4	155	389
9	195	7	84	408	*	*	*	*	172	4	115	305
10	280	7	160	579	*	*	*	*	193	4	50	325
11	307	7	92	652	*	*	*	*	316	4	222	472
12	170	7	89	373	*	*	*	*	154	4	103	233
13	198	6	95	396	*	*	*	*	139	4	87	236
14	108	7	53	235	*	*	*	*	103	4	92	119
15	173	7	101	300	*	*	*	*	174	4	106	305
	Evaluation Samples											
Unit/ Trailer No.	Formaldehyde				Acetaldehyde				Acetic Acid			
	Mean	n	Min	Max	Mean	n+	Min	Max	Mean	n	Min	Max
Remov (1)	353	34	112	552	4.2	14	3.2	5.8	187	14	103	284
Forever Fresh (2)	138	34	54	218	4.1	13	3.2	5.5	172	14	101	244
Safehome (3)	133	20	43	218	4.8	1	4.8	4.8	93	7	51	173
Control (4)	161	34	43	251	4.6	12	3.2	9.1	164	14	86	251
HEPAirX (5)	182	34	44	294	4.1	9	2.2	5.5	161	14	69	237
KES (6)	211	34	57	346	4.9	20	3.2	7.2	124	14	52	186
AirsoPure (7)	149	20	62	260	4.2	3	3.6	5.3	121	7	68	202
ANGUS Chem. (7)	190	14	82	249	4.6	10	3.2	5.5	127	7	50	239
Eraldehyde (8)	150	34	19	343	4.6	15	3.2	7.3	139	14	86	217
MaxxAir (9)	48	34	11	83	3.7	1	3.7	3.7	40	14	24	69
Fluid Lines (10)	169	34	55	266	10.9	30	3.6	18.1	84	14	34	142
Texas A&M (11)	351	17	85	544	7.1	15	3.6	10.6	220	6	136	288
Pureti (11)	432	17	195	562	9.7	17	5.5	12.8	203	8	148	303
Nanocepts (12)	95	34	25	139	5.7	25	3.6	8.8	71	14	24	133
Aria Acqua (13)	100	34	27	158	8.5	32	3.6	12.6	66	14	24	110
AirOcare (14)	112	34	33	199	4.0	18	2.8	5.4	89	14	23	135
Airxcel (15)	142	34	49	206	3.9	14	2.1	5.5	101	14	23	170

Table 6 continued. Summary concentration data (ppb) for formaldehyde, acetaldehyde, and acetic acid samples.

Trailer No	Formaldehyde				Acetaldehyde				Acetic Acid			
	Mean	n	Min	Max	Mean	n^+	Min	Max	Mean	n	Min	Max
					Post-evaluation Baseline Samples							
1	418	6	371	501	4.4	6	3.5	5.4	124	4	81	221
2	154	6	111	211	4.7	6	3.6	5.4	94	4	48	165
3	155	6	119	202	4.5	2	3.6	5.4	70	4	33	100
4	191	6	149	260	4.3	5	3.5	5.4	116	4	80	167
5	236	6	167	317	4.8	6	3.6	5.5	95	4	48	202
6	284	6	229	338	3.5	6	3.4	3.7	60	4	23	150
7	205	6	164	262	4.4	6	3.5	5.3	70	4	33	150
8	325	6	289	399	3.8	6	3.6	5.1	107	4	66	183
9	255	6	193	314	4.1	6	3.5	5.3	86	4	65	115
10	359	6	229	458	6.0	6	5.2	7.2	117	4	80	197
11	379	6	331	474	5.3	6	5.2	5.4	114	4	80	183
12	200	6	156	253	4.3	5	3.6	7.0	68	4	24	134
13	233	6	196	291	4.7	5	3.5	7.3	65	4	32	132
14	166	6	112	201	4.9	4	3.6	5.4	69	4	32	133
15	222	6	172	285	6.3	6	3.6	7.3	101	4	63	181

* All acetaldehyde baseline samples were non-detected. $^+$ Number of samples detected.

Air samples were collected and analyzed for VOCs by use of modified EPA method TO-17. During the baseline testing periods, 6 VOC samples were collected from each trailer, 4 during the pre-evaluation baseline sampling period, and 2 during the post-evaluation baseline sampling period. Seven samples were collected from each trailer during the device evaluation sampling period. Ambient air samples were also collected and analyzed for VOCs on the same days that sampling occurred in the trailers.

Table 7 identifies the compounds that were detected in each trailer and in ambient air during the pre- and post-evaluation baseline sampling periods as well as during the unit evaluation sampling period. Table 7 also provides mean concentrations for compounds whose concentrations were above 1–2 ppb and/or compounds found in all or most of the samples collected. It should be noted that many of the substances found were reported as "tentatively identified compounds" by the laboratory and that the concentrations for these particular compounds are reported as estimated values.

Table 7. Mean concentrations (ppb) of volatile organic compounds found above 1–2 ppb and/or compounds found in all or most of the samples collected during baseline and evaluation sampling. Checked items were detected but at low concentrations.

Analyte	Remov Trailer 1			Forever Fresh Trailer 2			Safehome Trailer 3			Control Trailer 4			HEPAirX Trailer 5		
	Pre	Test	Post	Pre	Test	Post	Pre	Test	Post	Pre	Test	Post	Pre	Test	Post
2-butanone (MEK) (J)	✓														
4-methyl-2-pentanone	✓										✓		✓		
2-methyl-butane															
acetaldehyde															
acetic acid (J)	140	32	31	28	30	47	44	13	17	30	32	39	56	29	44
acetone	2.2	1.0	5.3	2.0	3.7	1.8	2.1	2.2	2.0	2.0	1.9	4.3	4.0	2.5	6.0
acetonitrile															
α-pinene (J)	5.6	4.8	9.8	3.1	5.0	7.4	2.9	1.3	7.0	4.3	4.8	11	4.8	4.8	14
C7 alkene (J)										✓					
dibutyl phthalate (J)	✓			✓	✓		9.2	✓		9.4			✓	2.5	
dichlorodifluoromethane		✓	✓	✓	✓		✓	✓		✓			✓	✓	✓
ethanol			✓	✓			✓						✓		
formic acid (J)	15	1.2		2.0	1.6		✓			5.5			2.3	1.7	2.9
Freon 113	✓					✓									
hexanal (J)	2.0	2.2	2.7	2.0	2.2	2.3	✓		✓	✓	✓		2.7	1.6	1.4
isopropyl alcohol													✓		
methylene chloride	✓	✓	✓	✓			✓	✓	✓	✓	2.0	✓	2.4	✓	✓
nonanal (J)	2.5	3.8	3.4	2.5	4.2	3.5	2.2	1.0	2.8	1.0	2.2	2.7	2.4	2.6	4.0
pentanal (J)															
phenol (J)	1.4	✓		✓	✓		✓			✓		✓	✓	✓	✓
propanoic acid, 2-methyl (J)		1.0	1.1	1.2	1.4	2.7	1.0		1.0	0.2	0.2	1.2	1.3	0.2	1.3
styrene	✓		✓	✓		2.5		✓				✓	✓		2.0
tetradecane (J)	1.0	1.4	1.0	1.4	1.1	1.3	✓	0.2	1.1	1.1	0.4	1.3	1.0	0.5	1.4
toluene	✓												✓		
triacetin (J)				✓			✓								
tridecane	✓	✓	✓	✓			✓			✓					
xylene					✓										

Table 7, continued. Mean concentrations (ppb) of volatile organic compounds found above 1–2 ppb and/or compounds found in all or most of the samples collected during baseline and evaluation sampling. Checked items were detected but at low concentrations.

Analyte	KES Trailer Trailer 6			Airsopure Trailer 7			Angus Chem Trailer 7			Eraldehyde Trailer 8			MaxxAir Trailer 9		
	Pre	Test	Post	Pre	Test	Post	Pre	Test	Post	Pre	Test	Post	Pre	Test	Post
2-butanone (MEK) (J)				✓			✓			✓			✓		
4-methyl-2-pentanone										✓	✓				✓
2-methyl-butane															
Acetaldehyde				✓			✓								
acetic acid (J)	3.3	31	20	26	20	30	26	8.7	30	51	40	19	50	5.5	18
Acetone	1.7	3.0	18	2.0	1.8	5.7	2.0	3.9	5.7	2.3	5.1	2.0	3.3	2.2	2.4
Acetonitrile															
α-pinene (J)	2.5	3.2	7.2	4.4	8.4	10	4.4	2.0	10	4.1	4.5	8.0	4.8	0.6	14
C7 alkene (J)	✓			✓			✓								
dibutyl phthalate (J)	7.9	1.7		7.9	1.7		7.9	✓		✓	5.6		5.5	1.2	
Dichlorodifluoromethane	✓	✓	2.0	✓		✓	✓		✓		✓		✓	✓	
Ethanol	✓								✓			✓	✓	✓	✓
formic acid (J)				✓			✓			7.1			3.2	✓	
Freon 113															
Hexanal (J)	2.0	1.6	1.0	1.8	✓	1.0	1.8		1.0	2.6	2.4	1.4	2.1	0.4	2.7
isopropyl alcohol															
Methylene chloride	✓	✓	✓	✓		✓	✓		✓	✓			✓		6.9
Nonanal (J)	2.0	2.6	3.3	1.5	✓	3.0	1.5	1.0	3.0	2.4	2.6	4.4	2.2	1.4	4.7
Pentanal (J)										✓					
Phenol (J)	✓	✓		✓	✓	✓	✓	✓	✓	2.4	✓	✓	✓		
propanoic acid, 2-methyl (J)		0.7	1.5		1.6	2.9			2.9		✓	4.3	0.7		2.1
Styrene			✓	✓	✓	2.0	✓		2.0	✓	✓	✓		✓	✓
Tetradecane (J)	1.0	1.0	1.4	1.3	1.6	1.6	1.3	0.2	1.6	1.9	1.4	2.0	1.1	✓	1.1
Toluene				✓			✓			✓	✓				
Triacetin (J)													✓		
Tridecane		✓		✓			✓						✓		
Xylene				✓			✓	✓		✓					

Table 7, continued. Mean concentrations (ppb) of volatile organic compounds found above 1–2 ppb and/or compounds found in all or most of the samples collected during baseline and evaluation sampling. Checked items were detected but at low concentrations.

Analyte	Fluid Lines Trailer 10			Texas A&M Trailer 11			Pureti Trailer 11			Nanocepts Trailer 12			Aria Aqua Trailer 13		
	Pre	Test	Post	Pre	Test	Post	Pre	Test	Post	Pre	Test	Post	Pre	Test	Post
2-butanone (MEK) (J)	✓									✓			✓		
4-methyl-2-pentanone	✓			✓			✓	✓					✓		
2-methyl-butane															
Acetaldehyde				✓			✓				3.4				
acetic acid (J)	68	20	20	52	19	35	52	69	35	65	20	26	51	5.1	2.4
Acetone	2.5	18		2.3	12	6.2	2.3	10	6.2	3	19	1.6	1.5	18	
Acetonitrile				✓											
α-pinene (J)	3.6	3.3	14	✓	3.0	14	✓	9.6	14	3.5	1.4	7.9	5.1	3.8	6.5
C7 alkene (J)										✓			✓		
dibutyl phthalate (J)		✓		2.8	✓		2.8	2.1		1.4	1.1		3.7	✓	
Dichlorodifluoromethane	✓	✓		✓	✓					1.2	✓		✓	✓	✓
Ethanol	✓	✓	57	✓		✓		✓	✓	2.6	✓			✓	✓
formic acid (J)	4.5	✓	2.4	✓	4.6		✓	5.0		2.6	✓		6.3		
Freon 113															
Hexanal (J)	2.3	✓	3.0	2.7	1.1	2.9	2.7	3.1	2.9	2.1	✓	2.0	2.0	✓	✓
isopropyl alcohol						✓		✓	✓	✓	✓	2.1	✓	✓	2.7
Methylene chloride	✓	✓	5.9	✓	3.7	8.1	✓	✓	8.1	✓	✓	3.8		✓	12
Nonanal (J)	1.7	✓	5.2	2.0	1.8	4.0	2.0	4.7	4.0	2.4	✓	3.3	1.8	✓	1.7
Pentanal (J)		1.5													
Phenol (J)	✓			✓	✓					2.1	✓	✓	✓		
propanoic acid, 2-methyl (J)	1.4	✓	1.0	0.7	0.6	2.6	0.7	7.3	2.6	2.4	✓	2.9	✓	✓	✓
Styrene		✓	1.2	✓		1.6		1.8	1.6	✓		✓			✓
Tetradecane (J)	✓	✓	✓	✓	✓	1.3	✓	✓	1.3	✓	✓	1.3	✓	✓	✓
Toluene	✓	✓		✓									✓		
Triacetin (J)				✓											
Tridecane															
Xylene															

Table 7, continued. Mean concentrations (ppb) of volatile organic compounds found above 1–2 ppb and/or compounds found in all or most of the samples collected during baseline and evaluation sampling. Checked items were detected but at low concentrations.

Analyte	AirOcare Trailer 14			Airxcel Trailer 15			Ambient		
	Pre	Test	Post	Pre	Test	Post	Pre	Test	Post
2-butanone (MEK) (J)	✓			✓			✓		✓
4-methyl-2-pentanone				✓					
2-methyl-butane							✓	✓	
Acetaldehyde							1.4	✓	
acetic acid (J)	35	20	32	14	27	21	7.1	1.2	2.7
Acetone	1.9	2.9	✓	3.1	2.0	5.0	✓	✓	✓
Acetonitrile							11	2.1	8.9
α-pinene (J)	3.8	4.8	12	4.8	✓	14	✓		
C7 alkene (J)									
dibutyl phthalate (J)	5.5	✓			✓		4.4	✓	
Dichlorodifluoromethane	✓			✓	✓	✓	✓	✓	2.0
Ethanol		✓			✓	1.7		✓	1.8
formic acid (J)	2.0		2.4	2.2	2.6				
Freon 113									
Hexanal (J)	✓	✓	2.1	2.5	1.4	31	✓	✓	
isopropyl alcohol		✓				3.7			4.0
Methylene chloride	✓	✓	3.6			12		✓	17
Nonanal (J)	1.5	1.4	3.0	1.6	2.5	3.3	✓	✓	✓
Pentanal (J)									
Phenol (J)	✓			✓	✓	✓			
propanoic acid, 2-methyl (J)	1.1	0.7	4.8	✓	✓	2.9			
Styrene				✓	✓	3.2			
Tetradecane (J)	1.1	0.9	1.0	✓	✓	1.2	✓		
Toluene	✓			✓					
Triacetin (J)							✓		
Tridecane	✓				✓				
Xylene									

The effectiveness in reducing formaldehyde and acetic acid concentrations of the different mitigation solutions was determined in two different ways. The first method calculated a ratio of the test trailer to the baseline concentration, normalized for the control trailer. A daily ratio for each trailer was calculated by dividing the concentration in a particular trailer for a given day by its mean baseline concentration, including both the pre- and post-baseline measurements. Comparing the concentration to the average baseline concentration for that same trailer controls for between-trailer variability. To control for the day-to-day variability, the normalized ratios were calculated by dividing the daily ratios by the daily ratio for the control trailer. Equation 2 details these calculations.

$$\text{Normalized Ratio}_{X_T} = \frac{\text{Daily Ratio}_{X_T}}{\text{Daily Ratio}_{\text{Control}_T}} = \frac{\dfrac{C_{X_T}}{C_{X_{\text{Baseline}}}}}{\dfrac{C_{\text{Control}_T}}{C_{\text{Control}_{\text{Baseline}}}}} \tag{2}$$

Where: X = Trailer number, 1 to 15,

T = time,

$\text{Normalized Ratio}_{X_T}$ = control normalized ratio of trailer X at time T,

Daily Ratio_{X_T} = baseline normalized ratio of trailer X at time T,

$\text{Daily Ratio}_{\text{Control}_T}$ = baseline normalized ratio of control trailer at time T,

C_{X_T} = concentration in Trailer X at time T,

$C_{X_{\text{Baseline}}}$ = mean baseline concentration in Trailer X,

C_{Control_T} = concentration in Control Trailer at time T, and

$C_{\text{Control}_{\text{Baseline}}}$ = mean baseline concentration in Control Trailer.

A plot of these normalized ratios versus time for formaldehyde is given in Figure 2. Similar plots for acetic acid are given in Figure 3. For those samples taken in trailers that were non-detected (11 of 369 samples acetic acid, none for formaldehyde), concentrations were estimated from Equation 3[24]

$$m_{est} = \frac{EQL}{\sqrt{2}} \qquad (3)$$

Where: m_{est} = estimated sample mass, µg,

           EQL = estimated quanititation limit.

Note that the ratio for the control trailer is always 1.0, and a lower ratio implies a more effective strategy.

The second method for determining effectiveness calculated normalized mean ratios using Equation 4.

$$\text{Normalized Ratio}_{X_{Mean}} = \frac{\dfrac{C_{X_{Mean}}}{C_{X_{Baseline}}}}{\dfrac{C_{Control_{Mean}}}{C_{Control_{Baseline}}}} \qquad (4)$$

Where: $\text{Normalized Ratio}_{X_{Mean}}$ = control normalized average ratio of trailer X,

           $C_{X_{Mean}}$ = mean concentration in Trailer X, and

           $C_{Control_{Mean}}$ = mean concentration in Control Trailer.

This calculation provides an overall indication of the effectiveness of the different mitigation strategies; like the normalized ratios, it attempts to control for between-trailer and day-to-day variabilities. Note that the ratio for the control trailer is always 1.0 for both calculations and that a lower ratio implies a more effective control strategy.

44

A bar chart of the normalized average ratios for formaldehyde is given in Figure 4; the chart for acetic acid is given in Figure 5.

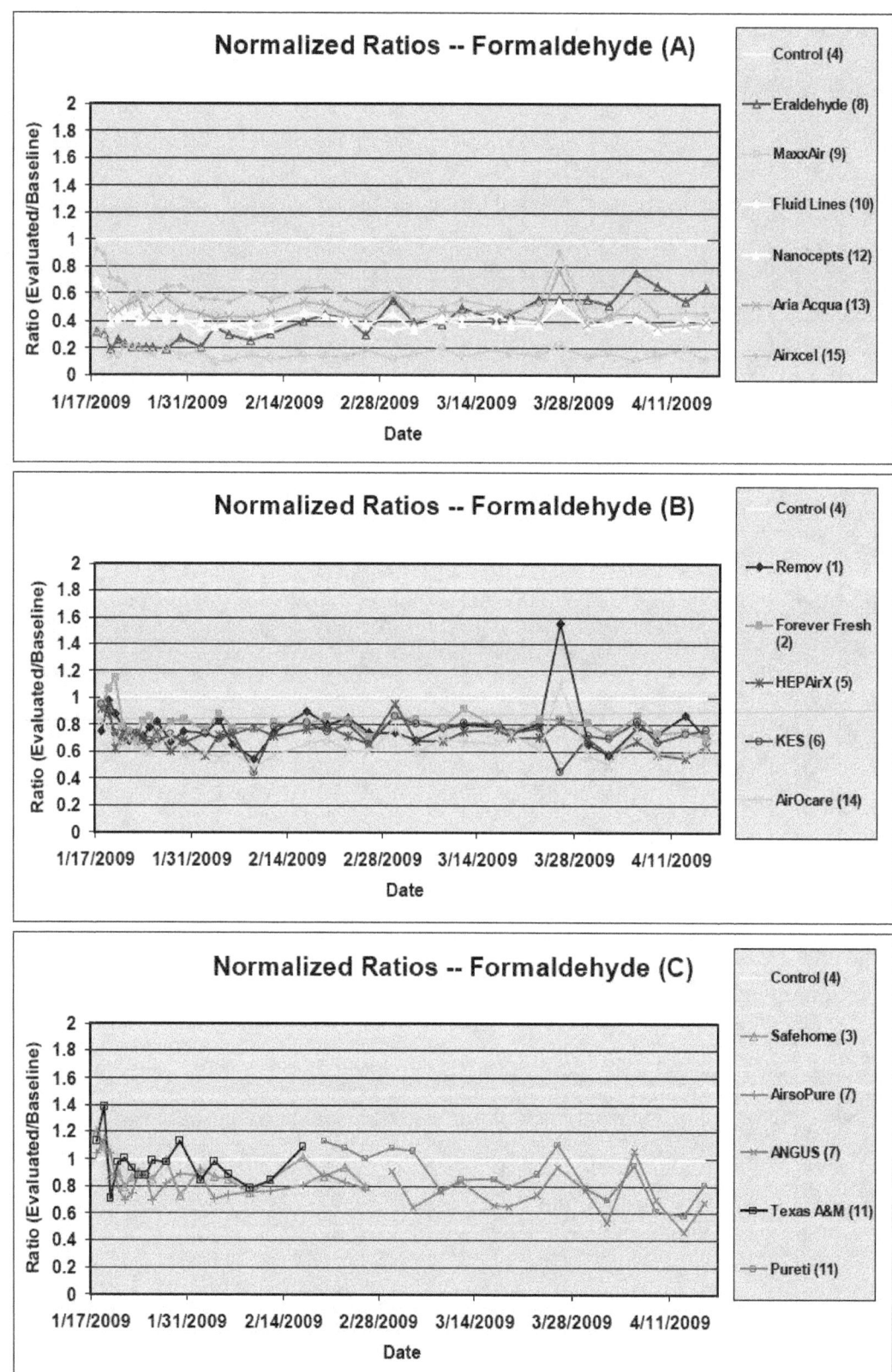

Figure 2. Plots of normalized ratios of technology evaluation samples to baseline samples versus time for formaldehyde. Numbers in parentheses indicate the trailer number where the technology was tested. A ratio of 1.0 would indicate no effect on formaldehyde concentrations. Number in parentheses indicates trailer number where device was evaluated.

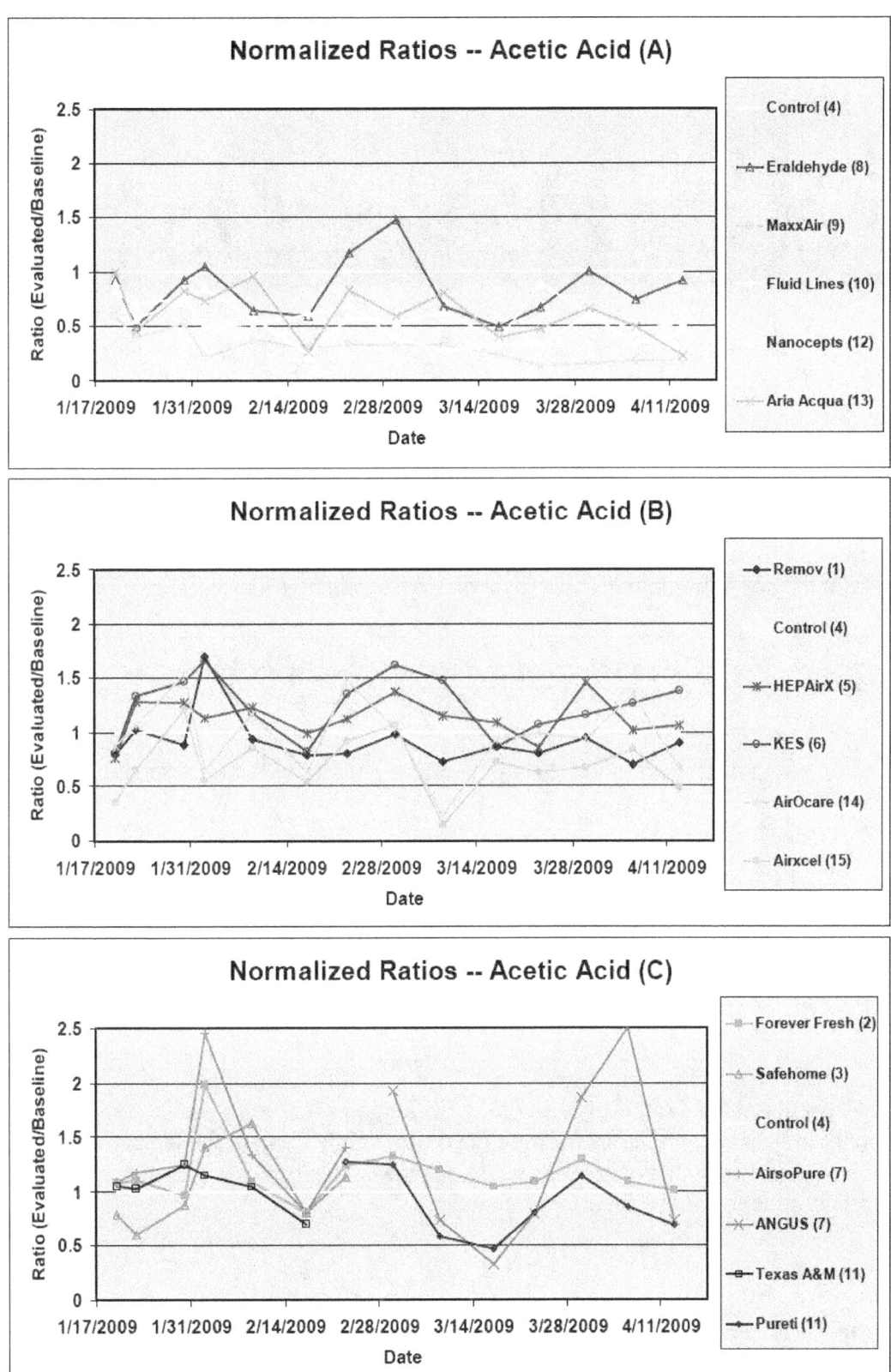

Figure 3. Plots of normalized ratios of technology evaluation samples to baseline samples versus time for acetic acid. Numbers in parentheses indicate the trailer number where the technology was tested. A ratio of 1.0 would indicate no effect on acetaldehyde concentrations. Number in parentheses indicates trailer number where device was evaluated.

47

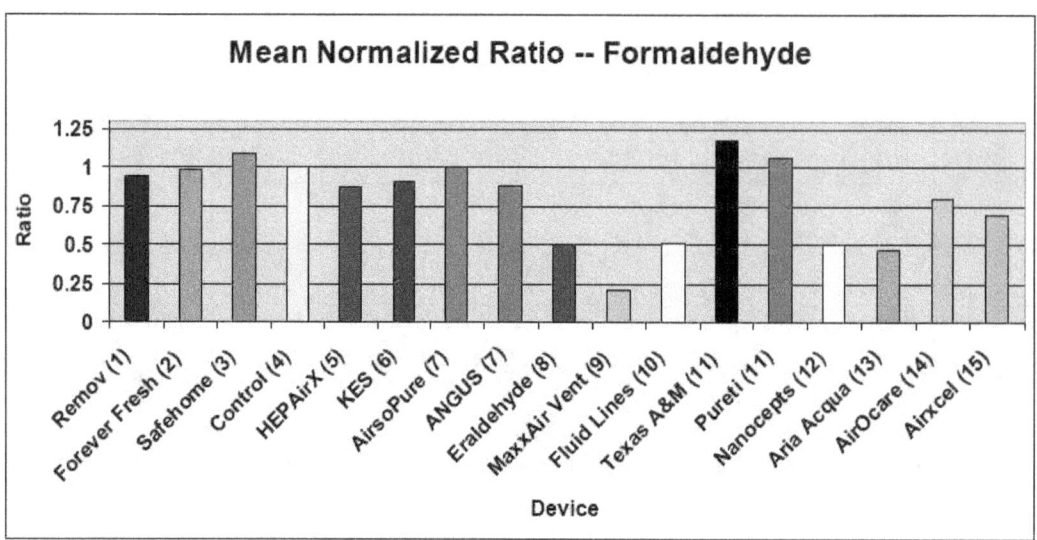

Figure 4. Mean normalized ratios of technology evaluation samples to baseline samples for formaldehyde. Numbers in parentheses indicate the trailer number where the technology was tested. A ratio of 1.0 would indicate no effect on formaldehyde concentrations. Number in parentheses indicates trailer number where device was evaluated.

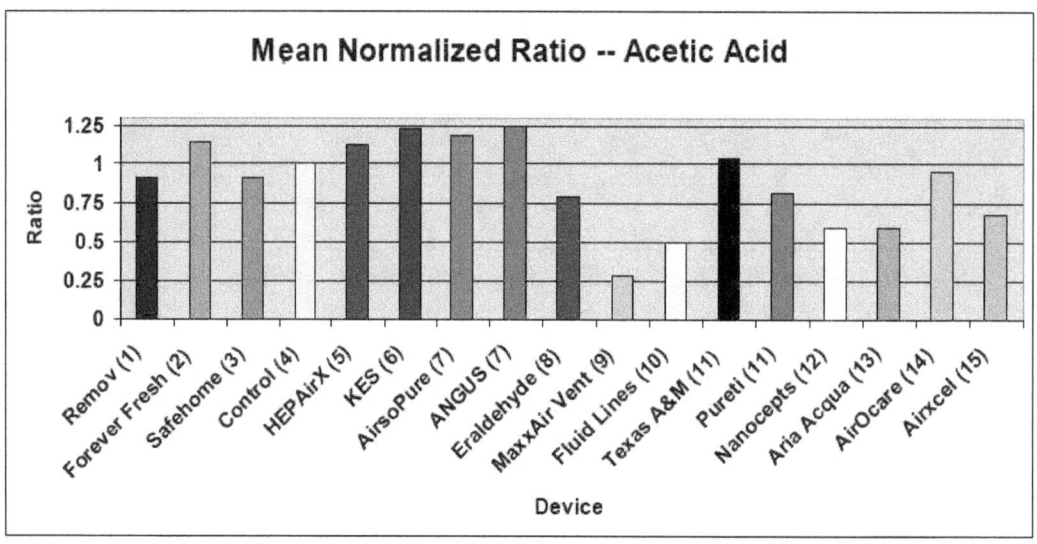

Figure 5. Mean normalized ratios of technology evaluation samples to baseline samples for acetic acid. Numbers in parentheses indicate the trailer number where the technology was tested. A ratio of 1.0 would indicate no effect on acetaldehyde concentrations. Number in parentheses indicates trailer number where device was evaluated.

While the ratios for acetic acid and formaldehyde provided a convenient means for assessing mitigation strategy effectiveness, a similar approach to the other compounds was not possible. As mentioned earlier in this report, the results of the TMPD-DIB sampling were all negative (not detected). In addition, for the aldehyde screening, only formaldehyde and acetaldehyde were detected. While the formaldehyde results were assessed with the calculation of the ratios, the concentrations of acetaldehyde was low relative to the limit of detection; in many cases, acetaldehyde was not detected. As all of the pre-evaluation baseline samples for acetaldehyde were below the analytical detection limit, a similar ratio could not be calculated. Table 8 provides information on the number of detected acetaldehyde samples during the evaluation and baseline sampling for each mitigation approach.

Table 8. Number and percentage of detected acetaldehyde samples. Baseline samples were all below the analytical limit of detection and are not included in the totals.

Technology (Trailer Number)	Evaluation Samples			Pre-Evaluation Samples			Post-Evaluation Samples		
	Total	Detect	Percent Detect	Total	Detect	Percent Detect	Total	Detect	Percent Detect
Remov (1)	34	14	41%	7	0	0%	6	6	100%
Forever Fresh (2)	34	13	38%	7	0	0%	6	6	100%
Safehome (3)	20	1	5%	7	0	0%	6	2	33%
Control (4)	34	12	35%	7	0	0%	6	5	83%
HEPAirX (5)	34	9	26%	7	0	0%	6	6	100%
KES (6)	34	20	59%	7	0	0%	6	6	100%
AirsoPure (7)	20	3	15%	7	0	0%	6	6	100%
ANGUS Chem. (7)	14	10	71%						
Eraldehyde (8)	34	15	44%	7	0	0%	6	6	100%
MaxxAir (9)	34	1	5%	7	0	0%	6	6	100%
Fluid Lines (10)	34	30	88%	7	0	0%	6	6	100%
Texas A&M (11)	17	15	44%	7	0	0%	6	6	100%
Pureti (11)	17	17	100%						
Nanocepts (12)	34	25	74%	7	0	0%	6	5	83%
Aria Acqua (13)	34	32	94%	7	0	0%	6	5	83%
AirOcare (14)	34	18	53%	7	0	0%	6	4	67%
Airxcel (15)	34	14	41%	7	0	0%	6	6	100%
Ambient	34	0	0%	7	0	0%	6	0	0%

9) DISCUSSION

This investigation was designed to explore the effectiveness of 16 devices at mitigating elevated formaldehyde concentrations. Efforts were made to control a number of different variables. This study design permits only limited analyses of the data. Although this evaluation assessed 16 different mitigation approaches, each was tested in only one trailer, yielding a sample size of one (n=1). Although many measurements of analyte concentrations were made for each approach, these measurements should be treated as repeated measures rather than as independent measurements. The value of one measurement may be dependent on the value of an earlier measurement. Considering these limitations, the results can provide an initial indication of the effectiveness of the tested approaches, thus forming the basis for a more definitive assessment of performance.

a. Temperature and Relative Humidity

The plots of the temperature data in Appendix E indicate that, with one exception, efforts to maintain a constant temperature in the trailers were reasonably effective as long as the outdoor temperature did not drop much below 2–5°C (35–41°F). While the set point for the heaters was 18°C (65°F), during colder days, the trailer temperatures could drop to below 15°C (59°F). Initially, two heaters were placed in the trailers. This resulted in numerous tripped circuit breakers, both in the trailers and at the main power supply panel for the trailers. Since upgrading power to the site was not an option and the trailers themselves had limited power options, the evaluation moved forward with one heater, limiting the ability to control lower temperatures. The high temperatures in the trailers appeared to be fairly well controlled with the trailers' air conditioning thermostats set to approximately 22°C (72°F). High temperatures in the trailers were maintained at approximately 24°C (75°F) or less.

51

The one exception to these observations on temperature was trailer 9, which contained the MaxxAir roof vent. This trailer had a much wider temperature swing at low outdoor temperatures, with the trailer temperature dropping as low as 2°C (35°F) when the outdoor temperature was -4°C (25°F). The 13.3 air changes per hour measured in the air exchange rate test (mean of two pre-evaluation and three post-evaluation tests) suggested that the MaxxAir unit exhausted 8.7 m^3/min (310 CFM). (Note that this unit was rated by the manufacturer at 27.8 m^3/min (982 CFM).) For each volume of air exhausted from the trailer, an equal volume of unconditioned air was brought in, through cracks in the trailer's envelop (i.e., cracks around doors and windows). It is clear that the large amount of air introduced into trailer 9 exceeded the space heater's capacity, with the result that temperature control was unreliable.

Relative humidity was monitored both in the trailers and outdoors. No attempts were made to control for humidity in the trailers. The plots of relative humidity with time, provided in Appendix E, indicate that, with the exception of trailer 9, the relative humidity in the different trailers was relatively consistent from one trailer to the next, although it did vary noticeably with time. Ambient relative humidity varied considerably more than in the trailers. The relative humidity in trailer 9 did not track the other trailers and can be attributed to the high ventilation rate from the MaxxAir unit.

b. Aldehdyes

In the development of the design of this evaluation, formaldehyde was the primary compound of interest. Because concerns existed that some of the technologies might generate a variety of contaminants, including other aldehydes, initial sampling and analysis included eleven other aldehydes besides formaldehyde (Table 2). As indicated earlier, only formaldehyde and acetaldehyde were detected in any of the samples, and the sample analysis was therefore scaled back to formaldehyde and acetaldehyde only for much of the evaluation.

During the pre-evaluation baseline sampling, acetaldehyde was not detected in any of the samples. During the evaluation sampling phase, acetaldehyde was detected in at least one sample from each of the trailers, including the control trailer. Table 8 provides the percentages of samples detected by trailer for each of the tested technologies. As shown in Table 6, the maximum concentration of acetaldehyde measured was 18 ppb. This data does suggest that certain technologies may produce more acetaldehyde than others. The three photocatalytic oxidation devices that were most effective in reducing formaldehyde concentrations (Fluid Lines, Aria Acqua, and Nanocepts) consistently had higher percentages of samples with detected levels of acetaldehyde. None of the ambient samples had detectable acetaldehyde concentrations.

The plots of the ratio of evaluation concentrations to baseline concentrations for the formaldehyde samples are shown in Figure 2. The mean ratios are shown in Figure 4. On the basis of these data, the MaxxAir system (Figure 2A), providing a mean 13.3 ACH, was the most effective unit, reducing formaldehyde concentrations by approximately 79%. This unit was a powered roof vent installed in the bathroom of the trailer. However, as indicated by the temperature and relative humidity data, operating this unit may result in less than optimal temperatures and relative humidities, and its use would likely result in a increase in energy consumption.

As mentioned earlier, the MaxxAir unit was a three-speed fan. The unit was evaluated at the highest fan speed, rated by the manufacturer at 27.8 m^3/min (982 CFM). This speed resulted in an actual ventilation rate of 8.7 m^3/min (310 CFM). The difference between actual and rated flow rates is likely due to the resistance the fan experiences during testing. While it is not explicitly stated in the product literature, the rated flow rate was likely measured with no resistance. With the fan installed in the trailer and all doors and windows closed, significant resistance for makeup air resulted in a lower actual flow rate. While this evaluation did not determine the formaldehyde concentrations during operation of the MaxxAir unit at the two slower fan speeds, 14.2 m^3/min (500 CFM) and 19.3 m^3/min (680 CFM), these concentrations can be predicted from the high fan speed data through a material balance, Equation 5.[25]

$$\text{Accumulation Rate} = \text{Generation Rate} - \text{Removal Rate}$$

$$V\,dC = G\,dt - \frac{QC}{K}\,dt \tag{5}$$

where: V = volume of enclosure, room, or trailer,

C = concentration at time t,

G = rate of generation of contaminant,

t = time

Q = rate of ventilation

K = mixing factor

Assuming G, K, and Q are constant, Equation 5 can be rearranged and integrated as shown in Equation 6.

$$\int_{C_{t_1}}^{C_{t_2}} \frac{dC}{G - \dfrac{QC}{K}} = \frac{1}{V}\int_{t_1}^{t_2} dt \tag{6}$$

where: C_{t_1} = concentration at time t_1

C_{t_2} = concentration at time t_2

Solving this integral and rearranging to solve for C_{t_2} yields Equation 7.

$$C_{t_2} = \frac{KG}{Q}\left[1 - e^{\left(\frac{-Q}{KV}(t_2 - t_1)\right)}\right] + C_{t_1} e^{\left(\frac{-Q}{KV}(t_2 - t_1)\right)} \tag{7}$$

As the system approaches equilibrium, (i.e., t_2 is large compared to t_1) the exponential term approaches 0, yielding Equation 8.

$$C_{t_2} \approx \frac{KG}{Q} \qquad (8)$$

For this calculation, we assume the mixing factor, K, and generation rate, G, will remain constant. It is further assumed that the fan's flow rate reduction due to resistance is proportional across the full range of flow rates. It is clear that the steady state concentration C_{t_2} is inversely proportional to the ventilation rate. Therefore, if the ventilation rate is cut in half, we would expect the concentration in the trailer to double. On the basis of Equation 8, operating the MaxxAir unit at the low fan speed would reduce formaldehyde concentrations by approximately 59%; at the medium setting, the reduction would be approximately 70%.

The Eraldehdye unit was nearly as effective as the MaxxAir unit during the first two weeks of operation; it reduced formaldehyde concentrations by 77%, compared to 79% for the MaxxAir in the first two weeks. These data are shown in Figure 2A. It should be noted that the performance of most of the units improved after the first 3 to 4 days of operation. The performance of the Eraldehyde unit began to diminish during the third week of operation, with a mean reduction during weeks three and four of 72%. Performance continued to decline in later weeks, with a mean reduction during weeks five and six of 62%, weeks seven and eight 55%, weeks nine and ten 51%, and weeks eleven through thirteen 39%. The Eraldehyde uses a treated filter to remove formaldehyde from the air. The treatment material appears to be rendered ineffective at a faster rate than anticipated. According to the manufacturer, this filter should last up to 6 months when used intermittently. In this evaluation, the unit was run continuously. The loss in effectiveness could be tied to a number of different causes. If the treatment material is being consumed at a fast rate, less material will be available to react with the formaldehyde. Dust loading of the filter could also be contributing. This unit uses a HEPA filter, and the collection of dust from the trailer would result in the formation of a filter cake. This filter cake could have an impact on the amount of formaldehyde in the air stream that actually contacts the reaction sites on the filter. Other unknown issues could also be playing a role in the diminished effectiveness of the Eraldehyde unit.

Figure 2A also shows the data for three prototype photocatalytic oxidation-based units, the Fluid Lines, Aria Acqua, and Nanocepts units. The performance of these three was very similar, resulting in formaldehyde concentration reductions of 50 to 55%. This level of performance remained fairly consistent throughout the test period. The final unit shown in Figure 2A was the AirXcel unit. This unit was a replacement air conditioning system that introduced a small amount of outside air into the trailer. On the basis of the air exchange rate tests in Tables 4 and 5, this system brought in about twice as much outside air, 1.03 ACH versus 0.511 ACH, than the same trailer with this outside air intake sealed. This system reduced formaldehyde concentrations by about 30%.

The performance of five units, AirOcare, HEPAirX, KES, Forever Fresh, and Remov, is shown in Figure 2B. The performance of five others, Safehome, ANGUS Chemical, Texas A&M, AirsoPure, and Pureti, is shown in Figure 2C. The AirOcare unit, based on an ionization technology, reduced formaldehyde concentrations by approximately 23%. The remaining units were marginally effective. None of these nine units (HEPAirX, KES, Forever Fresh, and Remov, Safehome, ANGUS Chemical, Texas A&M, AirsoPure, and Pureti) had removal rates in excess of 16%. The Texas A&M, AirsoPure, Safehome, and Pureti units appeared to have little if any impact on formaldehyde concentrations. The Texas A&M unit was removed from the test on February 18, 2009, due to inefficient formaldehyde removal performance, and it was replaced with the Pureti unit. The AirsoPure and Safehome units were similarly removed on February 27, 2009, and the ANGUS Chemical unit was installed in place of the AirsoPure unit.

Table 6 shows descriptive statistics for the baseline and evaluation samples. The formaldehyde concentrations in the trailers varied considerably during both baseline sampling periods and the evaluation sampling period.

c. Acetic Acid

The performance of the different technologies for reducing acetic acid, shown in Figures 3 and 5, is not as encouraging as the performance of the technologies for reducing formaldehyde. As in the case of formaldehyde removal, the MaxxAir unit showed the greatest reduction of acetic acid, at about 71%. The next most effective group was the PCO prototype units, the Fluid Lines, Aria Acqua, and Nanocepts devices, reducing acetic acid concentrations 50%, 41%, and 41%, respectively. The AirXcel unit had a reduction of 33%, similar to its 30% reduction for formaldehyde. The remaining units reduced concentrations by 25% or less, with six units having a mean normalized ratio of 1.0 or greater, indicating acetic acid concentrations were higher in the trailer when the unit was running than when it was not (figures based on the average of both pre- and post-baseline sampling).

d. 2,2,4-trimethyl-1,3-pentanediol di-isobutyrate (TMPD-DIB)

As all air samples for TMPD-DIB were below the analytical limit of detection, limited judgment can be offered as to the impact of the various technologies on the TMPD-DIB concentrations. The lack of detectable concentrations would suggest that none of the tested technologies generated significant quantities of TMPD-DIB.

e. Volatile Organic Compounds (VOCs)

As shown in Table 7, a substantial number of different VOCs were detected in the collected air samples. Acetic acid, α-pinene, and nonanal were found in every baseline and test phase indoor sample collected. Acetone, propanoic acid, and tetradecane were found in almost all indoor samples. Much lower levels (tenths to a few parts per billion) of these compounds were found in the ambient air.

With one possible exception, acetaldehyde, none of the oxidation technologies appeared to produce an intermediate product such as aldehydes, ketones, or acids over the course of the evaluation. The VOC sampling measured very little acetaldehyde; a single sample during the unit evaluation test period measured 28 ppb for the Nanocepts unit and three ambient samples were all below 3 ppb. However, numerous samples from the aldehyde screening were detected for acetaldehyde, as discussed earlier.

With the exception of formaldehyde and acetic acid, all other compounds present in the FEMA test trailers were within levels found in newly manufactured and site-built homes.[26] It should be noted that the manufactured homes tested by Hodgson et al. were 2- and 9-months old and that the testing was done 1–2 months after site-built homes were completed. The FEMA trailer mitigation air sampling occurred 3 years after the trailers were manufactured. Concentrations of airborne compounds in the trailers were likely higher in the past.

Table 9 displays the maximum contaminant concentrations of the most commonly found compounds (during technology and baseline testing), along with their respective odor thresholds, if available. Acetic acid and formaldehyde exceeded odor threshold values. Other compounds present (acetaldehyde, formic acid, propanoic acid, and styrene) also have pungent or sharp odors. The presence of the other compounds may increase the overall strength of odors and irritation effects indoors.

Table 9. Maximum concentrations during evaluation and baseline sampling with associated health-based screening guidelines and odor thresholds and characteristics.

Analyte	Maximum Concentration (ppb)		Health-based Inhalational Screening Guidelines	Odor Threshold (ppb) [26, 27]	Odor Characteristic [26, 27]
	Baseline	Evaluation			
2-butanone (MEK) (J)	3	3	2000[A]		
4-methyl-2-pentanone	4	2	700[A]		
2-methyl-butane	5	4			
Acetaldehyde–aldehyde	7.3	18.1	5[A]	186	Pungent/fruity
Acetaldehyde–VOC	5	28			
acetic acid (J)	424	127	10,000[B]	37–150	Pungent
acetone	84	84	10,000[B]	3600–65x10^4	Sweet/fruity
acetonitrile	29	9	36[A]		
A-pinene (J)	19	14		692	Pine
C7 alkene (J)	0	3			
dibutyl phthalate (J)	37	22			
dichlorodifluormethane	4	2			
ethanol	114	23			
formaldehyde	678	562	40[C]	500–1,000	Pungent
formic acid (J)	31	14			Sharp
Freon 113	0	1			
hexanal (J)	8	7		14	
isopropyl alcohol	8	16	3200[D]		
methylene chloride	33	15	300[E]		Sweet/etherish
nonanal (J)	6	10		2	
pentanal (J)	1	1			
phenol (J)	5	6	200[F]	110	
propanoic acid, 2-methyl (J)	6	12	10,000[B]		Sharp/pungent
styrene	4	3	200[E]	17-1900	Sharp/sweet
tetradecane (J)	2	4			
toluene	3	1	80[E]		
triacetin (J)	2	0			
tridecane	2	1			
xylene	6	6	50[E]		

Health Guidelines–[A]EPA Reference Concentration (RfC);[28] [B]NIOSH REL;[29] [C]ATSDR Acute MRL[30]; [D]CA Acute (1-hr) reference exposure level;[31] [E]ATSDR Chronic MRL;[30] [F]CA Chronic reference level exposure level.[31]

f. Assessing the Results Against Published Exposure Criteria

Table 9 also shows the available health-based guidelines, along with the maximum contaminant concentrations of all compounds detected during unit evaluation and baseline testing periods. Acetaldehyde and formaldehyde concentrations exceeded health-based guidelines. The maximum acetaldehyde concentrations during testing and baseline were 18 and 7 ppb, respectively. These values exceed the EPA's inhalation Reference Concentration (EPA RfC) of 5 ppb.[28]

Formaldehyde levels during unit evaluation and baseline sampling show maximum values of 562 and 678 ppb, respectively. These values exceed the American Conference of Governmental Industrial Hygienist (ACGIH) workers' short term (15-minute) exposure guideline of 300 ppb. Mean values during the unit evaluation and baseline sampling phases generally exceeded California's Acute Reference Exposure Level (REL) of 55 ppb in most samples in most of the trailers.

To understand the significance of the exposure criteria listed in Table 9, the following provides a brief discussion of each referenced criterion.

- An ATSDR Minimal Risk Level (MRL) is an estimate of the daily human exposure to a hazardous substance that is likely to be without appreciable risk of adverse non-cancer health effects over a specified duration of exposure. ATSDR health assessors and other responders use these substance-specific estimates, which are intended to serve as screening levels, to identify contaminants and potential health effects that may be of concern.

- ATSDR uses the no observed adverse effect level/uncertainty factor (NOAEL/UF) approach to derive MRLs for hazardous substances. They are set below levels that, based on current information, might cause adverse health effects in the people most sensitive to such substance-induced effects. MRLs are derived for acute (1–14 days), intermediate (>14–364 days), and chronic (365 days and longer) exposure durations.

- A California acute (1-hour) Reference Exposure Level (REL) is an estimate of the concentration level at or below which no adverse health effects are anticipated for a specified exposure duration. This concentration level is termed the reference exposure level (REL). RELs are based on the most sensitive, relevant, adverse health effect reported in the medical and toxicological literature. RELs are designed to protect the most sensitive individuals in the population by the inclusion of margins of safety. Since margins of safety are incorporated to address data gaps and uncertainties, exceeding the REL does not automatically indicate an adverse health impact.

- An EPA Reference Concentration (RfC) is an estimate of a continuous inhalation exposure for a given duration to the human population (including susceptible subgroups) that is likely to be without an appreciable risk of adverse health effects over a lifetime.

- A NIOSH time-weighted average (TWA) is a time-weighted average concentration guideline for occupational exposures up to a 10-hour workday during a 40-hour work week.

- A NIOSH short-term exposure limit (STEL) is a 15-minute occupational exposure guideline that should not be exceeded any time during the work week.

62

g. Study Limitations

While every effort was made to design the best evaluation possible, a variety of constraints have resulted in some limitations of the results. Most of the constraints are associated with the size and scope of the evaluation (e.g., number of trailers), while others are associated with variables that could not be well controlled (e.g., temperature and humidity). While the limitations may restrict generalizability of the results, the results do provide direction for decision-making concerning the application of mitigation formaldehyde strategies, including the need for further investigation.

For this evaluation, differences between different models of trailers were controlled by selecting test trailers that were as similar to each other as possible. The trailers were all built by the same manufacturer, in the same plant and on the same date. The limitation of this approach is that the results will be directly applicable only to these specific trailers. The findings may suggest that certain mitigation solutions could be effective beyond just these trailers, but the findings will not be definitive.

Changes in meteorological conditions are also a limitation. Formaldehyde generation from wood products is dependent, in part, on temperature and humidity. While the temperature within the travel trailers was controlled to a range, humidity was not directly controlled. Temperature and humidity measurements in the trailers were collected over the duration of field work. Because temperature and humidity could not be fully incorporated into data analysis, these results may not be valid outside the conditions present during field work. In addition, while the temperature within the trailer was held relatively constant, the temperature outside the trailer varied considerably, resulting in a varying temperature gradient across each trailer's envelop. The effect of this varying temperature gradient on formaldehyde emissions is unknown.

This evaluation assessed the effectiveness of the different technologies for a period of thirteen weeks. It is possible that some of the devices failed (e.g., malfunction or spent catalysts, chemicals, and absorption sites) during this period, but others functioned effectively throughout the entire test period. Failure modes and characteristics were not assessed for those that did function effectively for the entire time. While there was a screening of a wide variety of compounds during testing, it is possible that under real-world conditions, a particular device could fail in a manner not observed during this evaluation.

While this project attempted to evaluate the effectiveness of a variety of technologies for reducing formaldehyde concentrations in the travel trailers under controlled conditions, the effects of normal day-to-day activities by residents were not assessed. Activities such as cooking, smoking, and the use of cleaning products on the performance of the air cleaning devices could not be determined and could change the impact of some of the technologies or devices.

This evaluation assessed sixteen different devices. Although every effort was made to identify most of the primary categories of mitigation technologies for evaluation, other potential solutions may exist. In addition, the devices evaluated represented those specific units or technologies that were readily available either as commercial products or as working prototypes. Because of limited resources, testing of mitigation strategies were limited to assessing devices that do not generate ozone or UV light that could be seen by trailer occupants and that can easily be installed without significant trailer modifications. Ozone was a concern because of the respiratory health effects of ozone exposure. UV light was a concern because of possible ocular damage. Some strategies, such as treatments, were also eliminated from consideration due to the complexity and logistical challenges associated with implementation in the field.

Finally, this was not a statistical evaluation of technology effectiveness. The sixteen mitigation solutions were each evaluated in a single trailer, so that there was a sample size of one for each device. No statistical tests, calculation of confidence intervals, or other statistical methods were applicable, since there was no error term. Plots of concentration or efficiency versus time were generated for each device. Mitigation solutions that functioned well (for example, those that reduced formaldehyde concentrations to background levels for the duration of the evaluation) could be included in a future statistical study. Those that performed poorly, such as those having no impact on formaldehyde concentrations, could be omitted from future consideration.

10) CONCLUSIONS AND RECOMMENDATIONS

This evaluation assessed the effectiveness of sixteen different off-the-shelf or near-market-ready prototype devices for reducing formaldehyde concentrations in travel trailers used for temporary housing following disasters. The tested units included the following technologies: ventilation; oxidation, including photocatalytic oxidation, potassium permanganate, and two filter treatments; ionization; and adsorption. A primary objective was to determine if these mitigation devices were able to reduce the formaldehyde concentrations to a level that would be considered acceptable. An earlier CDC study of occupied travel trailers reported mean formaldehyde concentrations of 77 ppb, with a range of 3 to 590 ppb.[5] FEMA recently established a 16 ppb standard for new emergency housing.[32] For assessment purposes in this evaluation, these concentrations will be used to assess the effectiveness of the different mitigation devices at reducing concentrations to an acceptable level.

The MaxxAir unit, the powered roof vent, was the single, most effective unit evaluated. It resulted in a formaldehyde concentration reduction of approximately 79%. On the basis of the mean concentration of 77 ppb from the CDC occupied trailer study, installation of the MaxxAir vent would lead to a mean formaldehyde concentration of 16 ppb (79% of 77 ppb), the FEMA target concentration for new emergency housing. (Note: This calculation has no uncertainty term for the efficiency of the MaxxAir unit, and it uses a mean concentration from the CDC occupied trailer study; many of the tested trailers in the occupied trailer study tested at concentrations much higher than 77 ppb.) However, this unit exhausted 8.4 m³/min (300 ft³/min), representing 13.3 ACH, a high ventilation rate for a residence. The consequence of this high rate was demonstrated in the inability of the electric heaters to properly condition (heat) the trailer on the coldest days. On days where temperatures dropped to near freezing of lower, the heater was not able to maintain the set point temperature in the trailer with the MaxxAir unit installed. The effects of this high ventilation rate on either the factory-installed furnace or air conditioner are not known. However, the data do suggest that the use of this vent system would likely result in a substantial increase in utility use. The extent of that increase has not been determined and would depend upon ambient temperatures. In addition, the high ventilation rate in such a small occupied area would also likely result in drafty conditions in the travel trailer, particularly in the winter, further affecting the thermal comfort of the occupants. Finally, this device is configured with a speed selectable power switch, allowing the fan to be operated at any of three speeds or to be shut off. This device was evaluated at the highest fan speed and was operated continuously. If the MaxxAir device is installed in the travel trailers as a mitigation device, consideration should be given to removing the switch and installing the fan so that it runs continuously at the highest fan setting.

The Eraldehyde device had an initial performance that was very close to the performance of the MaxxAir vent. However, in less than a month, its performance deteriorated. This device removed formaldehyde from air by using a filter treated with a proprietary compound. It appears that the treatment compound was spent or rendered ineffective by dust loading or other unknown factors. The effectiveness of this unit might be maintained by frequent replacement of the treated filter, as frequently as once a month, assuming a formaldehyde generation rate similar to that of the test trailer. If the effectiveness of the Eraldehyde unit could be maintained to at least 70%, its use would result in mean concentrations of approximately 23 ppb (70% of 77 ppb), a figure based on the mean concentration of 77 ppb from the CDC study. While this concentration would not meet FEMA's target of 16 ppb, it does represent a significant improvement over the current circumstances.

Three prototype photocatalytic oxidation units, from Fluid Lines, Aria Aqua, and Nanocepts, all performed in a similar fashion, reducing formaldehyde concentrations 49% to 53% below baseline. All three of these units were relatively large, measuring approximately 0.3m x 0.46m x 0.76m (12" x 18" x 30"). These units would need to be reduced in size to be useable in the travel trailers. With a removal efficiency of approximately 50%, these units would result in mean concentrations of approximately 39 ppb (50% of 77 ppb), a figure based on the mean concentration of 77 ppb from the CDC study. This concentration would not meet FEMA's target of 16 ppb, although these units, used in conjunction with other technologies (as discussed later in this section), might reduce concentrations to an acceptable level.

One unit tested, the Airxcel unit, was an air conditioning system that incorporated a fresh air intake. This intake consisted of a hole drilled into the unit's return-air plenum and a small deflector to prevent the entry of water into the plenum. This unit reduced formaldehyde concentrations by approximately 30%. While this reduction would not achieve FEMA's target of 16 ppb, if installed in conjunction with other mitigation devices, it might prove to be acceptable. One advantage of this approach is that the existing air conditioning units could likely be modified to provide the needed fresh air. However, doing so would require the air conditioning fan to be run continuously, even during the heating season. The trailer's thermostat would need to be rewired to allow the fan to run at the same time as the trailer's furnace. Steps would need to be taken to ensure that such a configuration would not violate applicable codes or standards for the trailers.

The other devices tested in this evaluation proved to be only slightly effective or ineffective. None reduced formaldehyde concentrations by more than 20%, and in some cases, they resulted in no reduction. Even when used in conjunction with other, more effective devices, these units would likely not provide enough of a concentration reduction to justify their use.

Overall, there was no consistent decrease in VOC concentrations during the treatment technology test phase, compared to either the pre- or the post-baseline testing. In a few instances one VOC, but not all, decreased in a specific trailer. Likewise, a few instances of increases in VOCs occurred during the technology test period, but not with all VOCs in the specific trailer. Most differences between the baseline and testing phases were very small (e.g., 2 to 20 ppb) These small variations in concentrations likely were due to changes in temperature and, to a lesser extent, humidity during the different baseline phases and technology testing phase.

The use of multiple technologies might be an appropriate consideration for reducing formaldehyde concentrations to an acceptable level. For example, the Airxcel and Eraldehyde units (during the first 3–4 weeks of operation) were 30% and 70% effective, respectively. If these efficiencies are applied to the mean concentration of 77 ppb from the CDC occupied trailer study, the resulting mean concentration would be approximately 16 ppb ((1-.3) x [(1-.7) x 77 ppb] = 16 ppb), the FEMA target concentration for new emergency housing. Other combinations of technologies and units could be considered.

The primary contaminant of interest in this evaluation was formaldehyde; samples for other contaminants were collected, but none of the results showed concentrations above levels recognized to be of health concern. Some devices appeared to generate measureable concentrations of some compounds, such as several of the photocatalytic oxidations units that consistently generated detectable levels of acetaldehyde. However, these instances appeared to be limited, and concentrations of these compounds were low enough that they were not of toxicological concern. It is possible that byproducts for higher formaldehyde concentration environments may be higher. These byproduct compounds will, however, add to formaldehyde's eye, nose, and throat irritation effects. In addition, while the devices were screened for ozone and UV light emissions, some of these results would suggest a more comprehensive screening should be considered before any of these devices are deployed in occupied travel trailers. Any additional testing should include assessments of a similar array of compounds.

As stated in the DISCUSSION section of this report, the design of this evaluation has several limitations. A primary limitation resides in extending the results beyond the model of trailer used in the evaluation of the various mitigation devices. The results do suggest some possible courses of action that could reduce formaldehyde concentrations in occupied travel trailers. Any measures taken to reach the desired effectiveness (i.e., combining technologies or adopting one of the prototype technologies) should subsequently be evaluated in detail in a population of occupied travel trailers where these solutions are deployed. This step is needed to ensure that some unknown characteristic of the travel trailers in service will not have an adverse impact on the performance of the selected mitigation solution.

11) REFERENCES

1. Maddalena R, Russell M, Sullivan D, Apte M [2008]. Interim Report: VOC and Aldehyde Emissions In Four FEMA Temporary Housing Units, May 8, 2008. Lawrence Berkeley National Laboratory, Indoor Environment Department. Berkeley, CA

2. Recreation Vehicle Industry Association [2008]. About RVIA. [http://www.rvia.org/AM/ Template.cfm?Section=About_RVIA]. Date accessed: January 2008.

3. Sierra Club [2007]. Toxic Trailers? Tests reveal high formaldehyde levels in FEMA trailers. [http://www.sierraclub.org/gulfcoast/downloads/formaldehyde_test.pdf]. Date accessed: January 2008.

4. CDC/ATSDR [2007]. An update and revision of ATSDR's February 2007 health consultation: formaldehyde sampling of FEMA temporary-housing trailers. http://www.atsdr.cdc.gov/ substances/formaldehyde/pdfs/revised_formaldehyde_report_1007.pdf]. Atlanta, GA. Date accessed: January 2008.

5. NCEH [2008]. Final Report on Formaldehyde Levels in FEMA-Supplied Travel Trailers, Park Models, and Mobile Homes. Atlanta: U.S. Department of Health and Human Services, Public Health Service, Centers for Disease Control and Prevention, Coordinating Center for Environmental Health and Injury Prevention, National Center for Environmental Health. [http://www.cdc.gov/nceh/ehhe/trailerstudy/pdfs/FEMAFinalReport.pdf].Atlanta, GA. Date accessed: July 16, 2009.

6. 24 CFR 3280.308. Code of Federal regulations. Washington, DC: U.S. Government Printing Office, Office of the Federal Register.

7. EPA [2006]. Air Quality Criteria for Ozone and Related Photochemical Oxidents, Vol 1. EPA Report No. 600/R-05/004aF. U.S. Environmental Protection Agency, National Center for Environmental Assessment-RTP Office of Research and Development, Research Triangle Park, NC.

8. MaxxAir Vent Corp. [2009]. MaxxAir Turbo/Maxx. [http://www.maxxair.com/Products/Turbo-Maxx.aspx]. Tampa, FL. Date accessed: July 28, 2009.

9. Stevens L, Lanning JA, Anderson LG, Jacoby WA, Chornet N [1998]. Photocatalytic Oxidation of Organic Pollutants Associated with Indoor Air Quality, For Presentation at the Air & Waste Management Association's 91st Annual Meeting & Exhibition, June 14–18, 1998, San Diego, California, 98-MP9B.06.

10. MedicineNet, Inc [2008]. Definition of Reactive Oxygen Species. [http://www.medterms.com/script/main/art.asp?articlekey=26097]. Atlanta, GA. Date accessed: September 23, 2008.

11. AirOcare, Inc [2008]. AirOcare Clean Air Technology. [http://www.airocare.com/]. Rockville, MD. Date accessed: September 23, 2008.

12. No Odor, Inc [2008]. Cold Plasma. [http://www.noodor.net/id51.htm]. Fort Lauderdale, FL. Date accessed: September 29, 2008.

13. SilverMedicine.org [2008]. Ozone Generators—Medical and Therapeutic Grade Ozone Equipment. [http://www.silvermedicine.org/ozone-therapy-generators.html]. Las Vegas, NV. Date accessed: September 29, 2008.

14. Aerisa, Inc [2008]. Aerisa The Science of Clean Air. [http://www.aerisa.com/]. Scottsdale, AZ. Date accessed: September 29, 2008.

15. Filt Air Ltd. [2008]. Bi-polar Ionization with Sterionizer. [http://www.sterionizer.com/Sterionizer_Background.aspx]. Israel. Date accessed: September 29, 2008.

16. Clean Air Group, Inc [2008]. Atmosair—bi-polar ionization, clean air purification. [http://www.atmosair.com/how-it-works/atmosair-clean-air-technology.html]. Fairfield, CT. Date accessed: September 29, 2008.

17. Air Fantastic, LLC [2008]. Air Fantastic™ Quadruple Ion Technology. [http://www. airfantastic.com/what_is_photo.htm]. Austin, TX. Date accessed: September 30, 2008.

18. EPA [1999]. Compendium Method TO-11A, Determination of Formaldehyde in Ambient Air Using Adsorbent Cartridge Followed by High Performance Liquid Chromatography (HPLC). U.S. Environmental Protection Agency, Cincinnati, OH.

19. EPA [1999]. Compendium Method TO-17, Determination of Volatile Organic Compounds in Ambient Air Using Active Sampling Onto Sorbent Tubes. U.S. Environmental Protection Agency, Cincinnati, OH.

20. OSHA [1999]. Method PV2002, 2,2,4-Trimethyl-1,3-Pentanediol Diisobutyrate. U.S. Occupational Safety and Health Administration, Washington DC.

21. Edie, P [2008] U.S. Occupational Safety and Health Administration Methods Development Team, Industrial Hygiene Chemistry Division, Personal Communication September, 9 2008. OSHA Salt Lake Technical Center, Salt Lake City, UT.

22. NIOSH [2003]. Method 1603, Acetic Acid. NIOSH Manual of Analytical Methods. National Institute for Occupational Safety and Health, Centers for Disease Control and Prevention, Cincinnati, OH.

23. ASTM International [2006]. Standard test method for determining air change in a single zone by means of a tracer gas dilution.

24. Hornung RW, Reed LD [1990]. Estimation of average concentration in the presence of nondetectable values. Appl Occup Environ Hyg 5(1):46–51.

25. NIOSH [1973]. The Industrial Environment—Its Evaluation and Control. National Institute for Occupational Safety and Health, Cincinnati, OH.

26. American Industrial Hygiene Association [1989]. Odor Thresholds for Chemicals with Established Occupational Standards. Fairfax, VA.

27. ATSDR [1999]. Toxicological Profile for Formaldehyde. Atlanta, GA. U.S. Department of Health and Human Services, Centers for Disease Control and Prevention, Agency for Toxic Substances and Disease Registry.

28. EPA [2009]. Integrated Risk Information System (IRIS). U.S. Environmental Protection Agency. [http://www.epa.gov/iris/]. Date accessed: August 24, 2009.

29. NIOSH [2005]. Pocket guide to chemical hazards. Cincinnati, OH: U.S. Department of Health and Human Services, Centers for Disease Control and Prevention, National Institute for Occupational Safety and Health, DHHS (NIOSH) Publication No. 2005-149. [www.cdc.gov/niosh/npg/]. Date accessed: July 14, 2009.

30. ATSDR [2008]. Minimal Risk Levels (MRLs) for Hazardous Substances. Atlanta, GA. U.S. Department of Health and Human Services, Centers for Disease Control and Prevention, Agency for Toxic Substances and Disease Registry. [http://www.atsdr.cdc.gov/mrls/]. Date accessed: August 24, 2009.

31. OEHHA [2008]. Acute, 8-hour and Chronic Reference Exposure Levels (chRELs). Sacramento, CA. Office of Environmental Health Hazard Assessment, California Environmental Protection Agency. [http://oehha.ca.gov/air/allrels.html]. Date accessed: August 24, 2009.

32. FEMA [2008]. FEMA: New FEMA Procurement Specifications Require Significantly Reduced Formaldehyde Levels In Mobile Homes And Park Models. Washington, DC: U.S. Department of Homeland Security, Federal Emergency Management Agency. News Release: HQ-08-056, April 11, 2008. [http://www.fema.gov/news/newsrelease.fema?id=43180]. Date accessed: July 16, 2009.

APPENDIX A

OZONE AND UV LIGHT EMISSION TESTING METHODS AND RESULTS

Ozone Testing

All powered air purification devices being considered for this evaluation were assessed for ozone emissions. Units relying solely on ventilation or those relying on diffusion were not tested. A portable Ozone Monitor (2B Technologies, Inc.; Model # 205; Serial #: 635DB) was used to assess ozone omission; the instrument provided concentration measurements in ppb. For evaluation purposes, all devices were operated according to manufacturers' instructions. At the time of testing, ambient room temperature was approximately 22°C (72°F).

Before testing, background concentration measurements of ozone were made in the laboratory where the ozone testing was taking place. After recording the laboratory background concentration, the mitigation units' ozone emissions were measured. The sampling tube of the ozone monitor was placed approximately at 10–20 cm from the major output air stream of each device. Sampling from the output air stream occurred for approximately 10 minutes, allowing ozone generation (if ozone was being generated) to stabilize and reach a steady state. At this point, the ozone concentration reading was recorded.

The results presented in Table A-1 show all of the devices tested and the resultant ozone produced. Units that produced significantly elevated ozone levels (highlighted in grey) were excluded from the evaluation and returned to the originator.

Table A-1. Ozone emission test results for air purification units. Gray shaded devices were not evaluated in the test trailers due to high ozone output. Pink shaded devices were not evaluated in the test trailers due to high UV light output.

Device	Company	Technology	Back-ground Concen-tration (ppb)	Unit Concen-tration (ppb)
Formal X	So-Brite Chemicals International, Inc.	Treated Filter	Not Tested	
Forever Fresh	Worldwide Sales, Inc.	Passive diffusion/ adsorption	Not Tested	
Prototype	Safehome	Potassium Permanganate	4.9	1.1
HEPAiRx	Air Innovations	Ventilation	Not Tested	
AiroCide Ser No ACKS-251-111940	KES	Photocatalytic Oxidation	5.1	3.3
AiroCide Ser No ACKS-251-111893	KES	Photocatalytic Oxidation	6.2	3.3
S900 Ser No 000032	Airsopure	Photocatalytic Oxidation	6.2	5.0
S900 Ser No 000033	Airsopure	Photocatalytic Oxidation	6.5	3.9
Prototype	ANGUS Chemical	Treated Filter	1.8	2.4
Eraldehyde MODEL 802	MicroSweep Corp	Treated Filter	4.9	1.2
MaxxAir Turbo/ Maxx™ - 3550	Maxxair Vent Co.	Ventilation	Not Tested	
Prototype	Fluid Lines	Photocatalytic Oxidation	3.9	3.0
Prototype	PURETi	Photocatalytic Oxidation	3.1	1.5
Prototype Unit #1	Texas A&M University	Photocatalytic Oxidation	5.5	4.6
Prototype Unit #2	Texas A&M University	Photocatalytic Oxidation	3.8	3.3
Prototype	Nanocepts	Photocatalytic Oxidation	3.9	2.2
Prototype	Aria Acqua	Photocatalytic Oxidation	Not Tested	
Prototype	AirOcare	Reactive Oxygen Species	1.0	7.9
Coleman-Mach Air Conditioner	Airxcel, Inc	Ventilation	Not Tested	
Nanobreeze, Unit #1	NanoTwin Technologies	Photocatalytic Oxidation	5.4	10.5

Nanobreeze, Unit #2	NanoTwin Technologies	Photocatalytic Oxidation	6.9	10.3
Prototype	ActiveTek	ActivePure Technology (H_2O_2)	4	115.9
AF1000, Ser No. 008011	Air Fantastic	Quadruple Ion Technology	6.7	287.9
AF1000, Ser No. 002813	Air Fantastic	Quadruple Ion Technology	4.9	305.5
AFMini, Ser No. 008033	Air Fantastic	Quadruple Ion Technology	4.9	745.4
AFMini, Ser No. 008031	Air Fantastic	Quadruple Ion Technology	5.5	459.3
Prototype	AERISA	Cold Plasma	4.4	42.8
AtmosAir T-400 Ser No. 401107MTG1220	Clean Air Group	Bipolar Ionization	3.5	892.6
AtmosAir T-400 Ser No. 401107MTG1227	Clean Air Group	Bipolar Ionization	5.1	1297
AirOCare, Ser No 0033, with screen[*]	AirOcare	Reactive Oxygen Species	5.5	88.5
AirOCare, Ser No 0033, no screen[*]	AirOcare	Reactive Oxygen Species	5.5	61.6
AirOCare, Ser No 0034, with screen[*]	AirOcare	Reactive Oxygen Species	3.4	115.5
AirOCare, Ser No 0034, no screen[*]	AirOcare	Reactive Oxygen Species	3.4	82.5

[*] According to the manufacturer, a "screen' was provided with this unit to improve air cleaning. The unit could be operated with or without this screen.

UV Testing

The photocatalytic oxidation air cleaning units were evaluated for UV light emissions due to the use of a UV light source as a fundamental component of their oxidation process. UV light emissions were measured on those units where the UV light source was visibly exposed. Five units of three different models were assessed. An Ocean Optics Spectroradiometer (HR2000+ Spectrometer) was used to measure UV irradiance from UV-PCO units that had visually exposed light bulbs. An integrating sphere (~ 5 cm diameter) was attached to the input fiber optic of the Ocean Optics spectroradiometer, enabling the spectroradiometer to function as a cosine receptor irradiance sensor. A quartz-tungsten-halogen lamp (FEL #523) calibrated by Optronics Laboratories against a National Institute of Standards and Technology (NIST)-calibrated FEL lamp served as a calibrated irradiance source for the spectroradiometer. The input port of the integrating sphere was placed as close as possible to the UV source of each unit being tested. (Note: the placement of the integrating sphere at a point closest to the source represents a worst-case scenario in which the user of these devices would get as close to the UV source as possible without disassembling the unit.) A measurement of the light spectrum was performed. The spectroradiometer output was then converted to spectral irradiance through the NIST traceable calibration, and the spectral irradiance was integrated over the UV-A, UV-B, and total UV spectral regions.

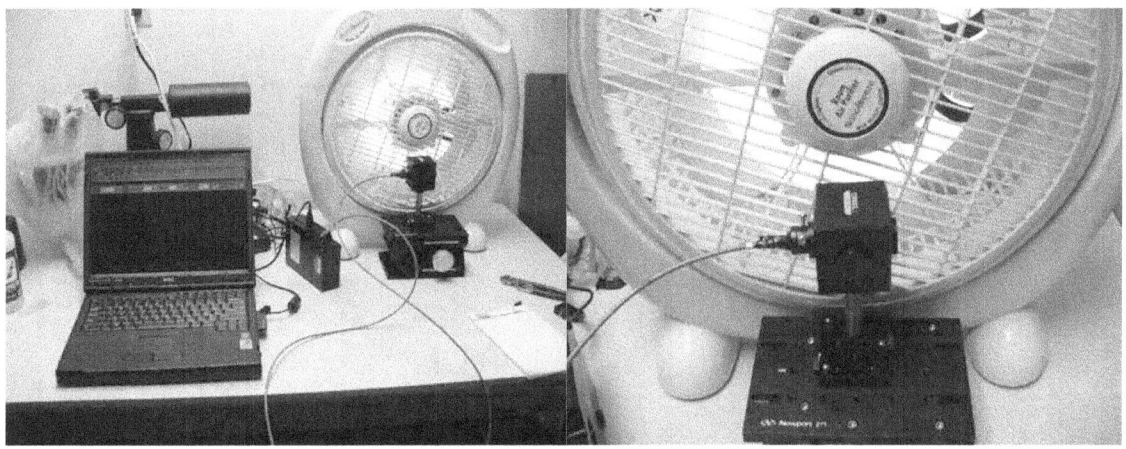

Figure A-1. Equipment configuration for measuring UV light emissions.

The spectral irradiance of Ultraviolet (UV) light wavelengths lie just below the short end of the visible spectrum (below 400 nm), and they are the most energetic and destructive form of light. UV radiation exposure is known to cause serious human health issues, like conjunctivitis, keratitis, and cataracts of the eye and skin erythema. UV radiation is divided into three distinct bands: UV-A, UV-B, and UV-C. Each has different penetration properties and potential for damage. The UV-A and UV-B bands were the focus of these measurements.

The American Conference of Governmental Industrial Hygienists (ACGIH) has published a Threshold Limit Value (TLV®) for occupational exposures to UV light. This TLV provides duration of exposure per day for a given Effective Irradiance for a broadband source. Table A-2 provides the spectral irradiance measurements and TLV durations for the Effective Irradiance measured for each device. The two tested Nanobreeze units had durations of less than 30 sec for their measured Effective Irradiance, while the other three devices had durations of 9.7 to 14 minutes. While all these measurements present a concern for the safety of users, the Nanobreeze units present a more acute concern because of the very short allowable exposure duration.

Table A-2. Results of UV emission testing for photocatalytic oxidation units. Pink shaded devices were not evaluated in the test trailers due to high UV light output.

Device/Company	Measured Irradiance UV-A (315–400 nm)	Measured Irradiance UV-B (280–320nm)	Effective Irradiance (Total) (280–400nm)	ACGIH TLV® Duration[*]
S900 Ser No 000032/ Airsopure	0.032 w/m2	0.018 w/m^2	0.047 w/m^2	14 min
S900 Ser No 000033/ Airsopure	0.035 w/m^2	0.020 w/m^2	0.053 w/m^2	9.7 min
Prototype/ PURETi	0.032 w/m^2	0.017w/m^2	0.046 w/m^2	14 min
Nanobreeze, Unit #1/ NanoTwin Technologies	1.848 w/m^2	0.061w/m^2	1.898 w/m^2	21 sec
Nanobreeze, Unit #2/ NanoTwin Technologies	1.493 w/m^2	0.058 w/m^2	1.541 w/m^2	25 sec

[*] Based on total UV measurement.

[A]   ACGIH [2009]. 2009 TLVs® and BEIs®. American Conference of Governmental Industrial Hygienist, Cincinnati, OH.

APPENDIX B

PHOTOGRAPHS OF MITIGATION UNITS AS DEPLOYED IN

THE TRAVEL TRAILERS

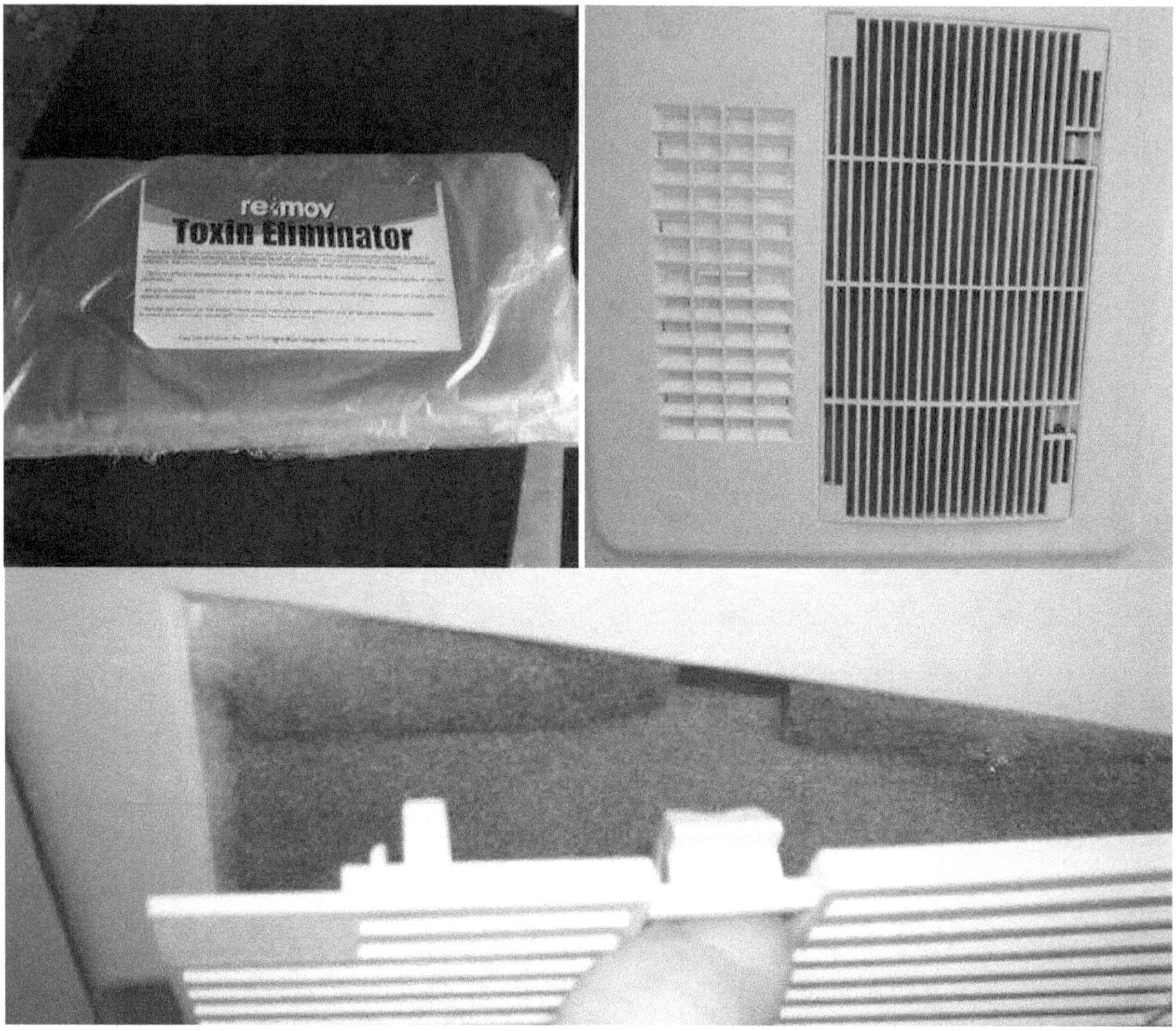

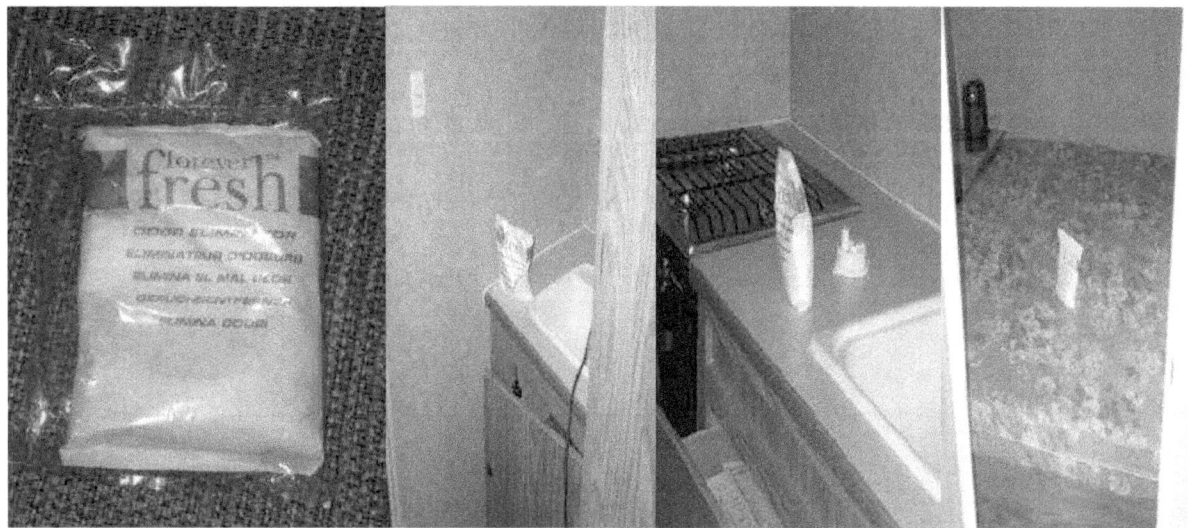

Figure B-1. Remov filters placed in Trailer 1.

Figure B-2. Forever Fresh placed in Trailer 2.

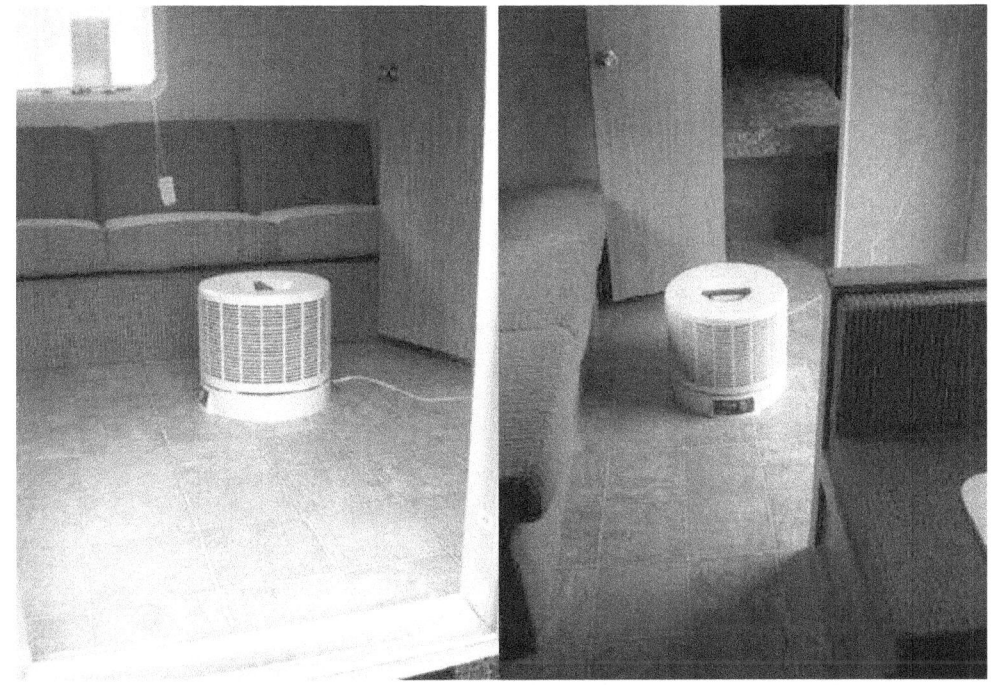

Figure B-3. Safehome device placed in Trailer 3.

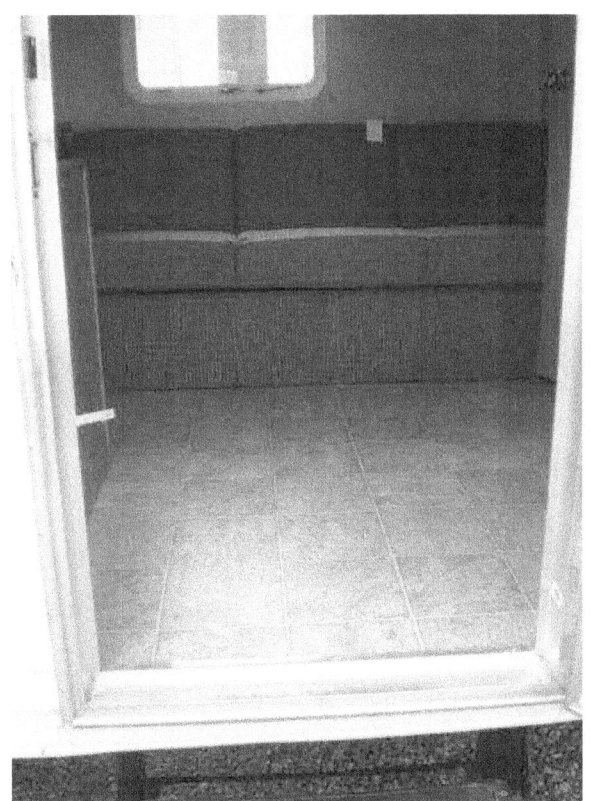

Figure B-4. Control, Trailer 4.

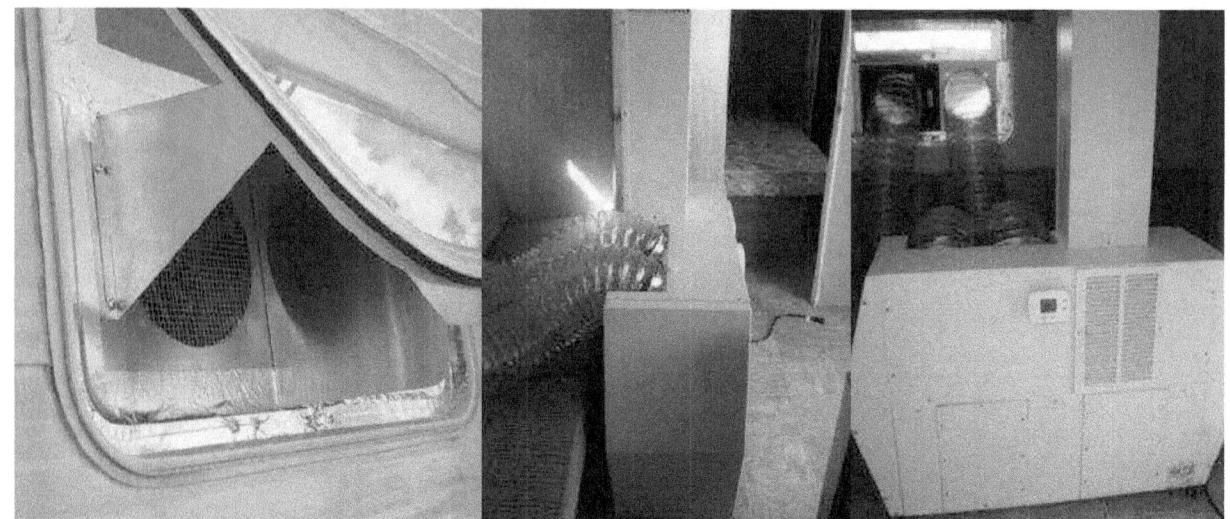

Figure B-5. HEPAiRx unit placed in Trailer 5.

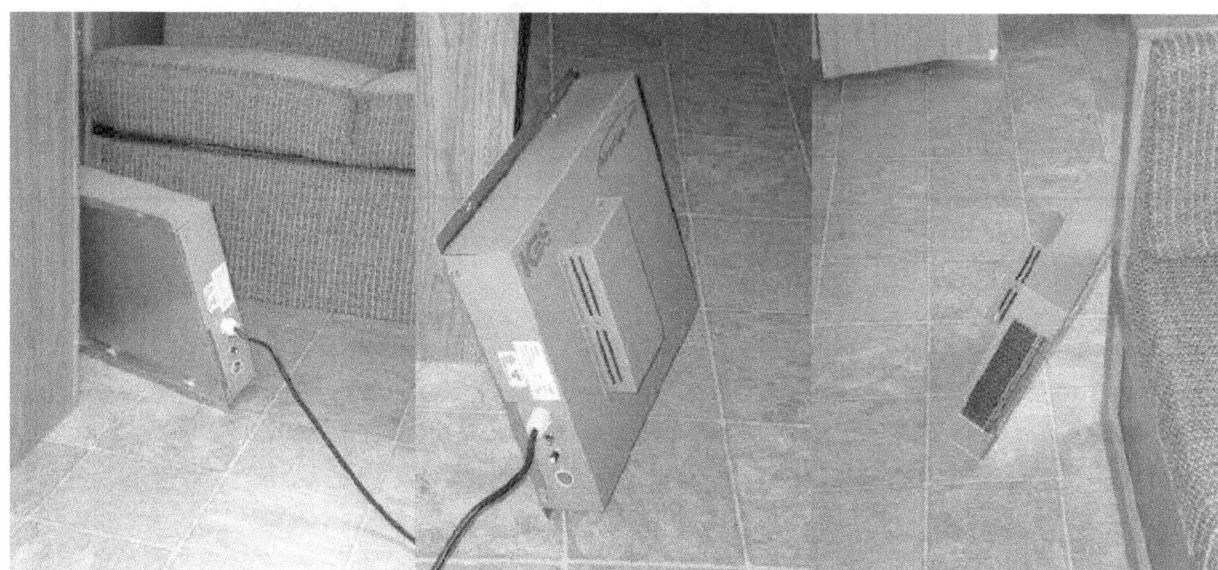

Figure B-6. KES/AiroCide unit placed in Trailer 6.

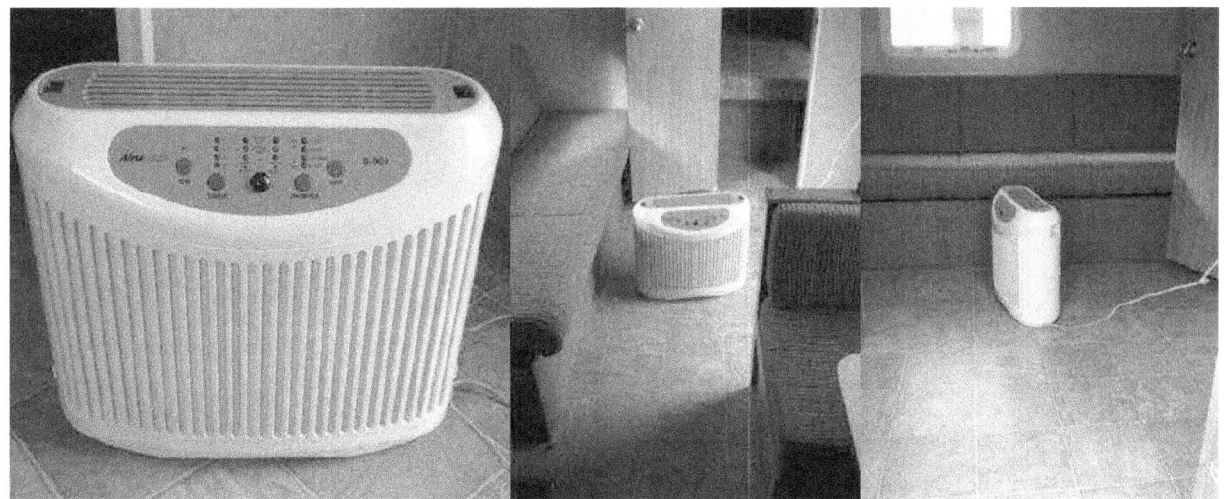

Figure B-7. AirSoPure S900 unit placed in Trailer 7.

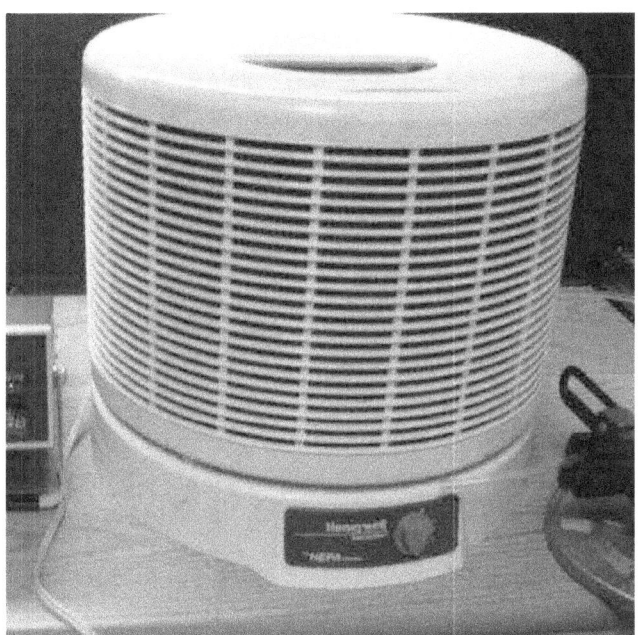

Figure B-8. ANGUS unit. Unit is not pictured as deployed in Trailer 7.

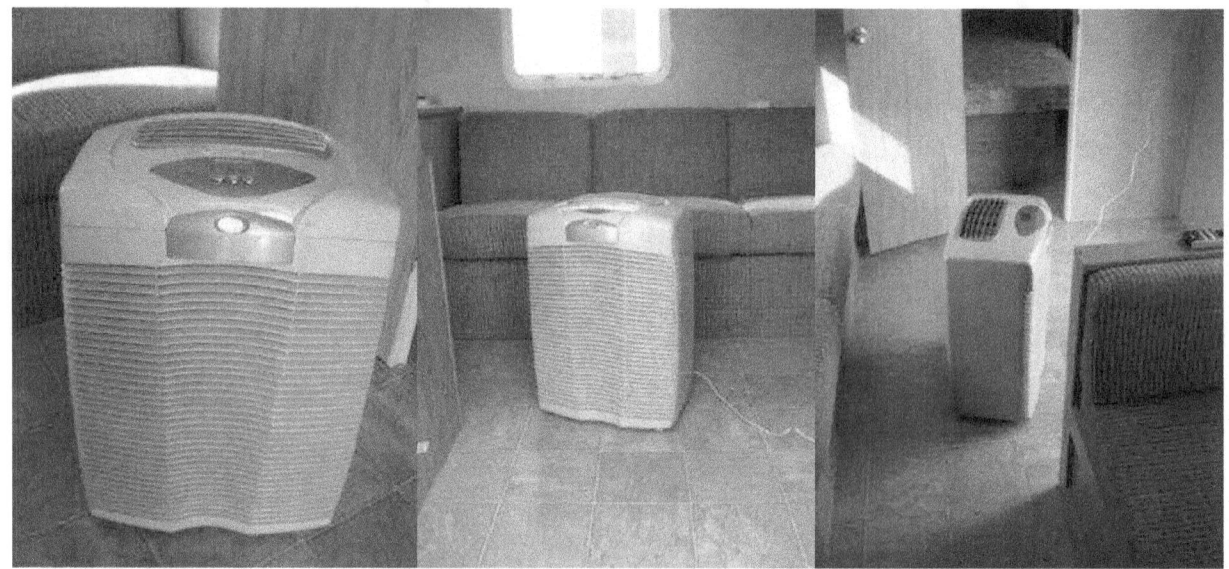

Figure B-9. Eraldehyde unit placed in Trailer 8.

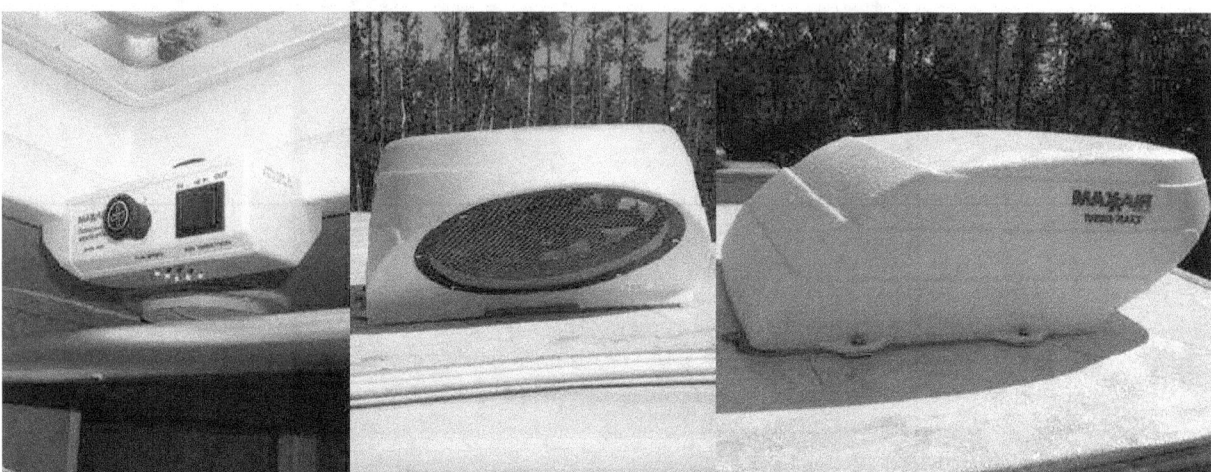

Figure B-10. MaxxAir unit installed in Trailer 9.

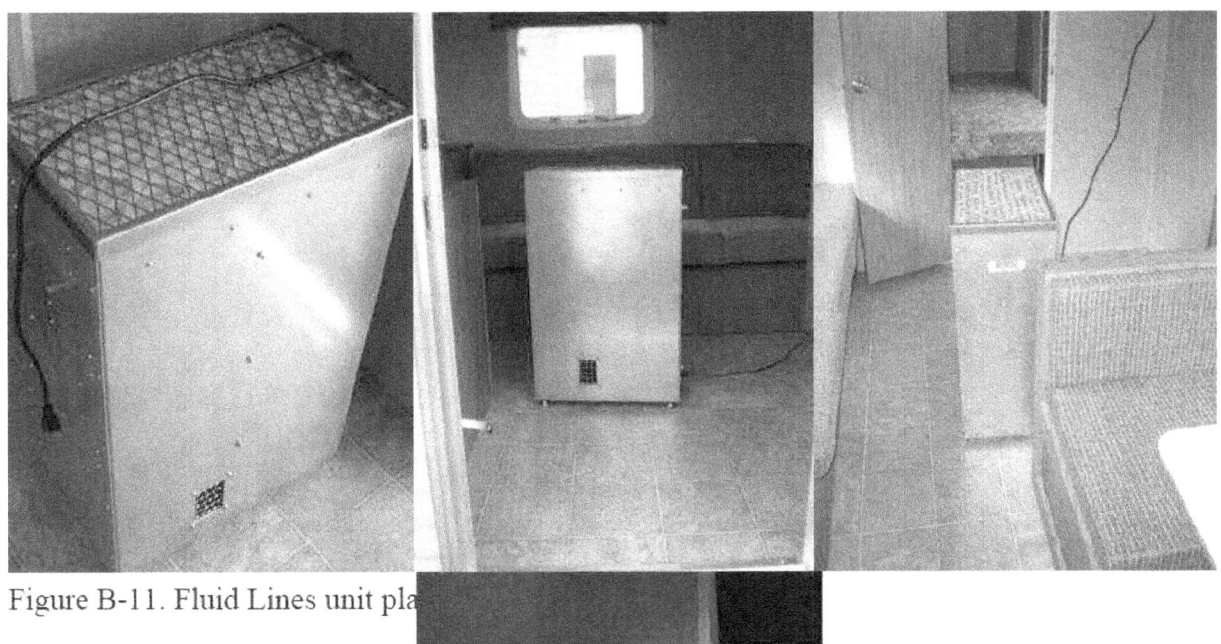

Figure B-11. Fluid Lines unit pla[...]

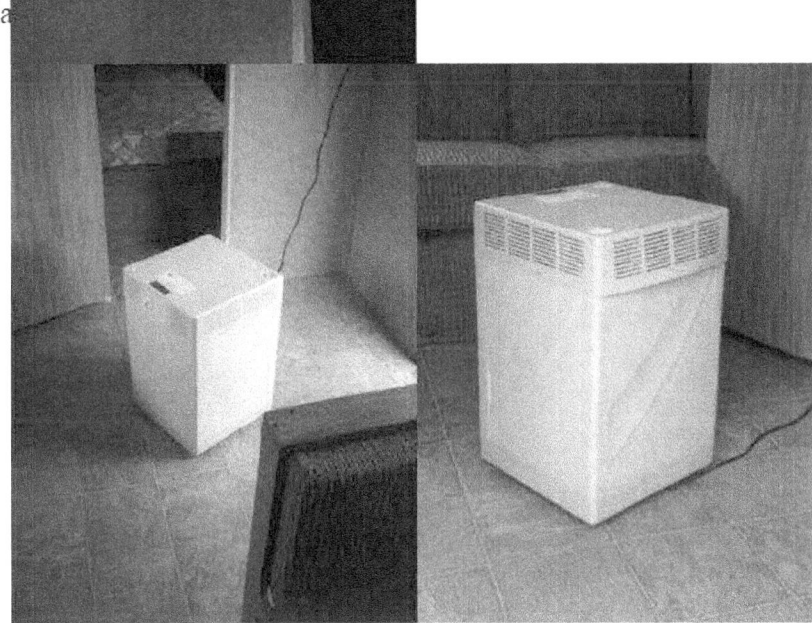

Figure B-12. Texas A&M unit placed in Trailer 11.

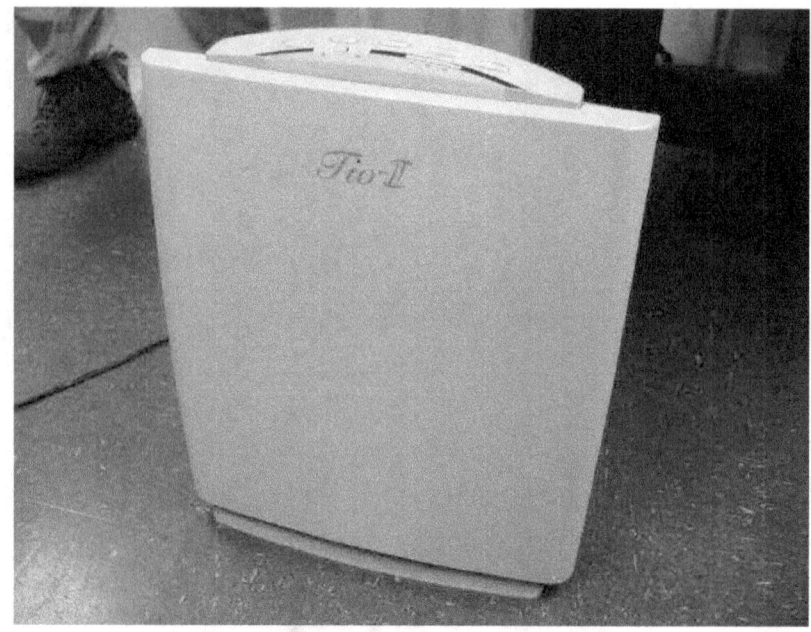

Figure B-13. Pureti unit. Unit is not pictured as deployed in Trailer 11.

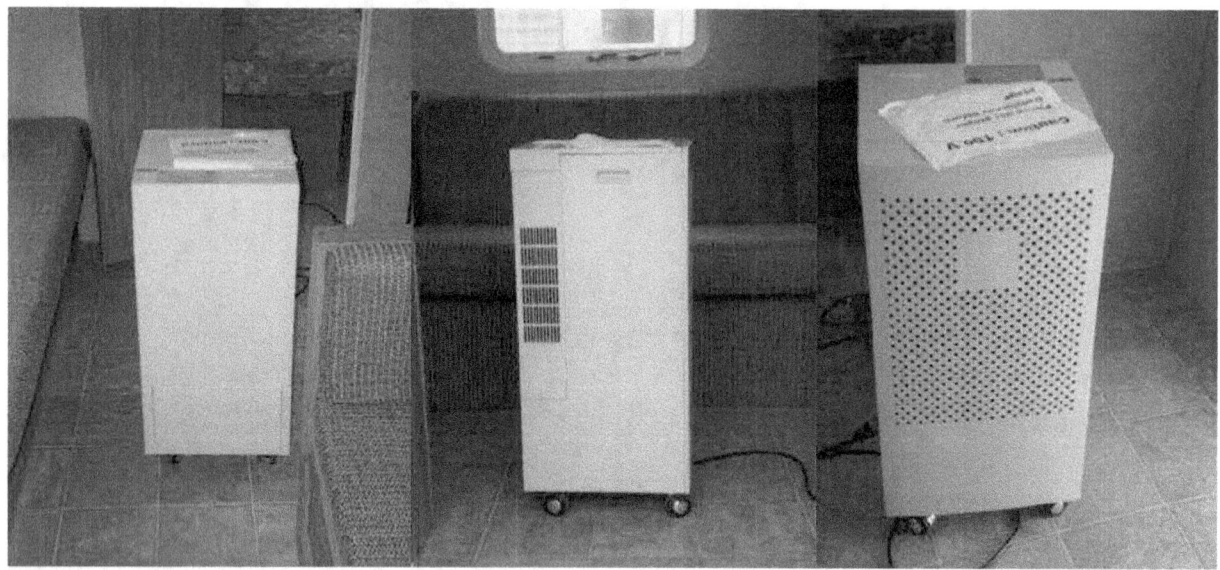

Figure B-14. Nanocepts unit placed in Trailer 12.

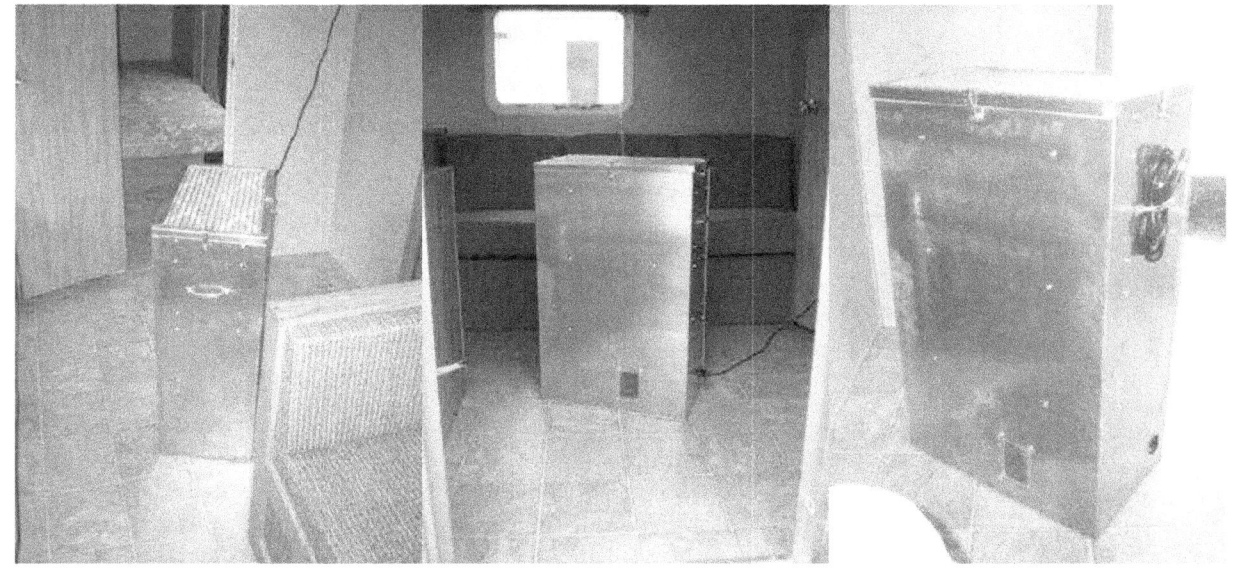

Figure B-15. Aria Acqua unit placed in Trailer 13.

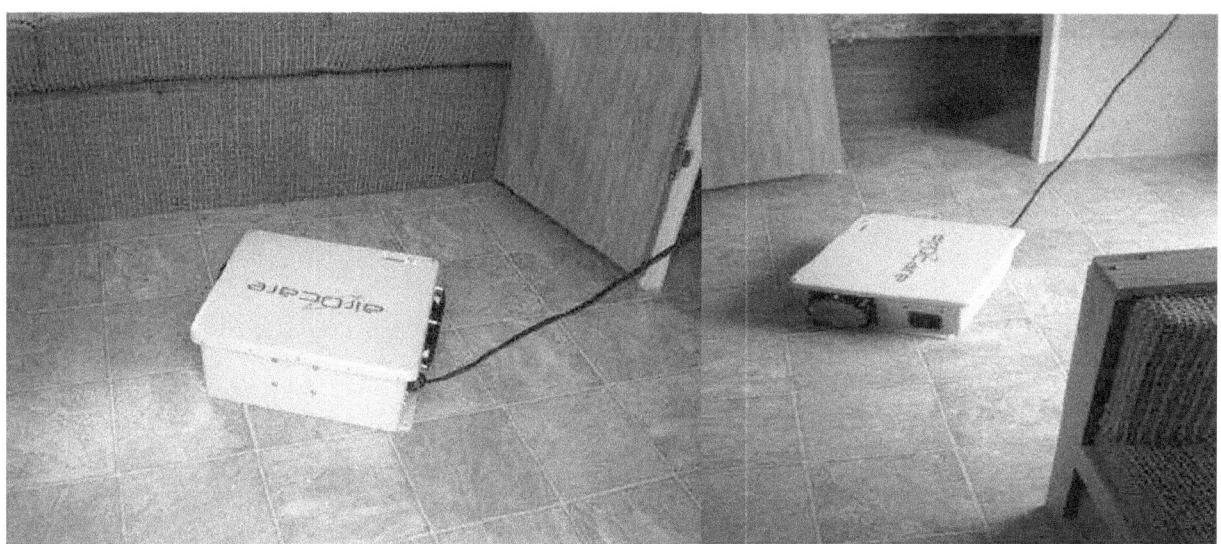

Figure B-16. AirOcare unit placed in Trailer 14.

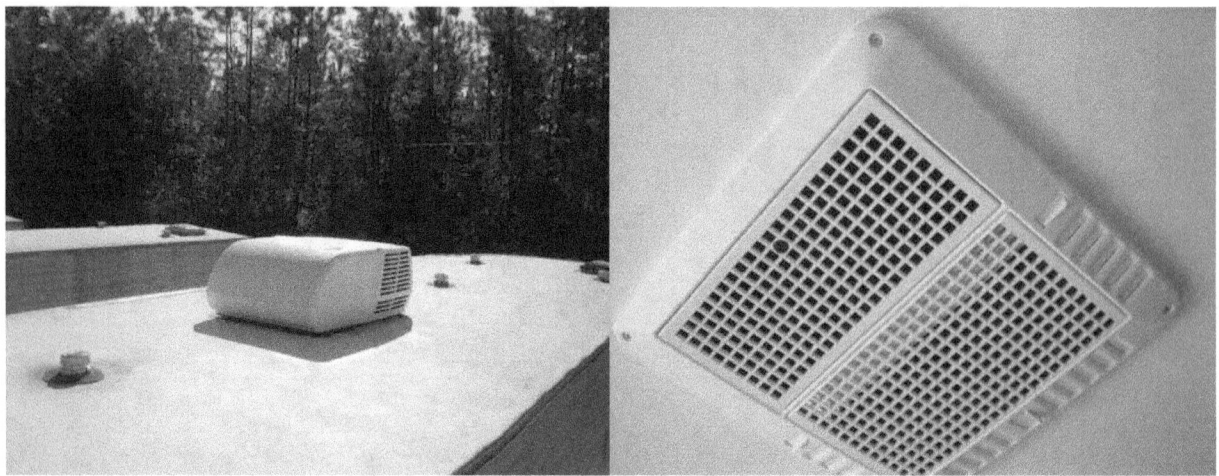

Figure B-17. AirXcel unit installed in Trailer 15.

APPENDIX C

AIR SAMPLING and QUALITY ASSURANCE/QUALITY CONTROL

Sample tube storage:

Sample tubes will be stored in a freezer or in coolers with ice/ice packs before and after sampling and during shipment.

Sampling pump calibration

Sampling pumps will be pre-and post-calibrated with a primary standard. The sampling pumps will be configured to operate on AC power, rather than batteries, for improved pump reliability. AC power will be available through receptacles located on the outside of the trailers. Pre- and post- calibration will be performed at the site where the trailers are staged.

Media blanks

Six to ten (or additional if required by the lab) media blanks will be collected from each lot of sample tubes used. Two to three blanks will be selected from the beginning, middle, and end of a lot. Media blanks will remain in packaging and not be opened. They will be labeled, logged on the chain of custody, and shipped the same day they were collected.

Field Blanks

Field blank samples will determine if field conditions or sampling techniques were conducted without artificially introducing chemical contamination. One blank sample will be collected for each sample media type used that day. Field sample blanks will be handled in a similar manner as the trailer samples, with the same numbering scheme and sample storage. Field sample blanks will be removed from any packaging, the medial opened (caps removed, ends of tubes broken, etc.). The tubes will be resealed and placed near the actual sampling tubes. Field sample blanks will be collected at the end of the sampling day. At this point, the field sample blanks are removed, sealed, and stored just like the trailer samples.

Documentation

All sample collection and chain of custody sheets are located in Appendix D. The sample collection data sheet will be used to record sample start and finish times, pump/instrument calibration, etc., by trailer. The survey data sheet includes information about download files for temperature and humidity. A data sheet will be filled out for each trailer on each sampling day. A completed sample chain of custody form will accompany each sample shipment to the laboratory.

Sample Shipment

Samples will be shipped overnight, on ice, to the laboratory. Except for Saturday, samples will be shipped at the end of each sampling day. There is no laboratory sample receiving activity on Sundays.

APPENDIX D

DATA SHEETS

Sample Collection Sheet

Sample Date: _____   Trailer Number*: _____   Samples Collected _____

by:

	Sample number	Tube Lot	Pump S/N	Calibrator S/N	Pre-sample calibration flow (ml/min)	Post-sample calibration flow (ml/min)	Average flow rate (ml/min)	Start time 24-HR FORMAT	Stop time 24-HR FORMAT
Formaldehyde Sample									
Volatile Organic Compound									
TMPD-DIB Sample									
Acetic Acid Sample									

* Assigned trailer number (1–15) or Field Sample Blank number (Blank1, Blank2)

Notes/observations:

APPENDIX E

TEMPERATURE AND RELATIVE HUMIDITY PLOTS

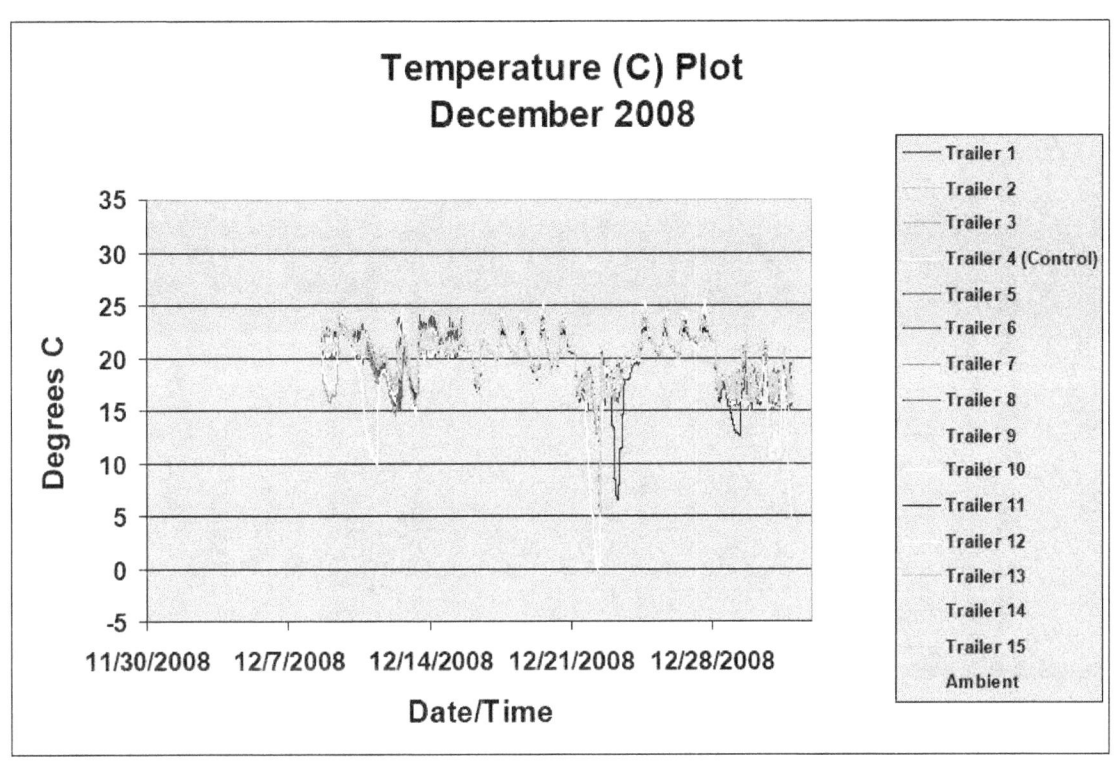

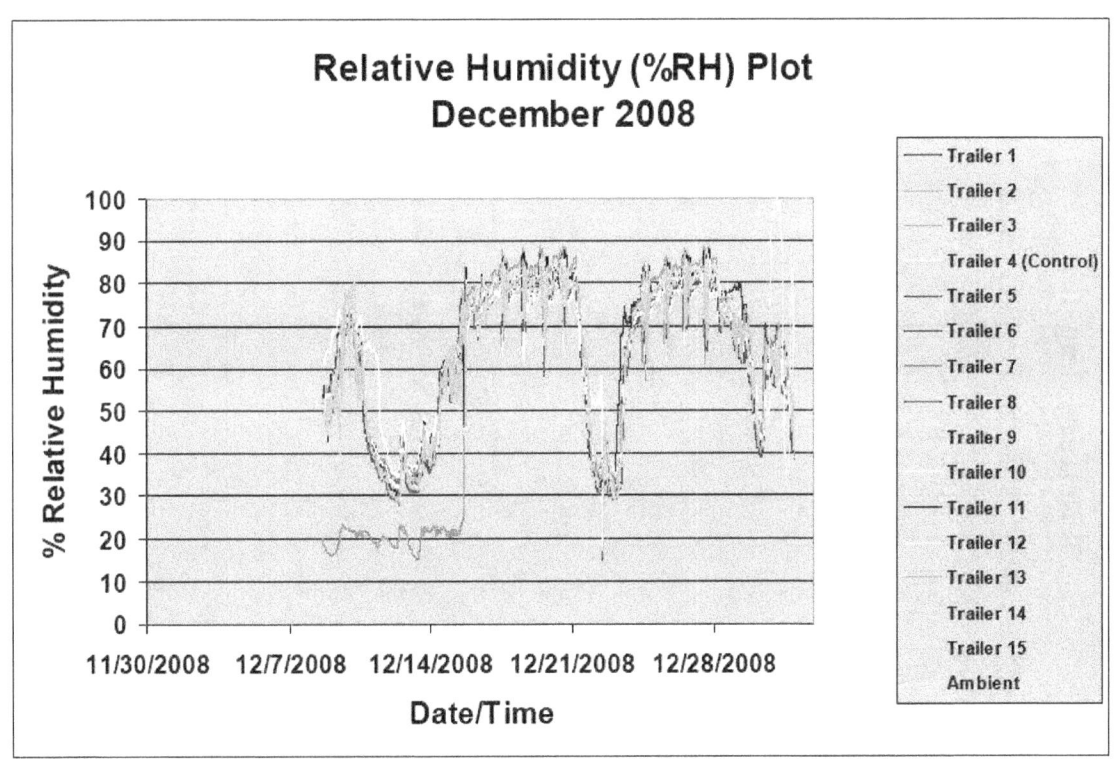

97

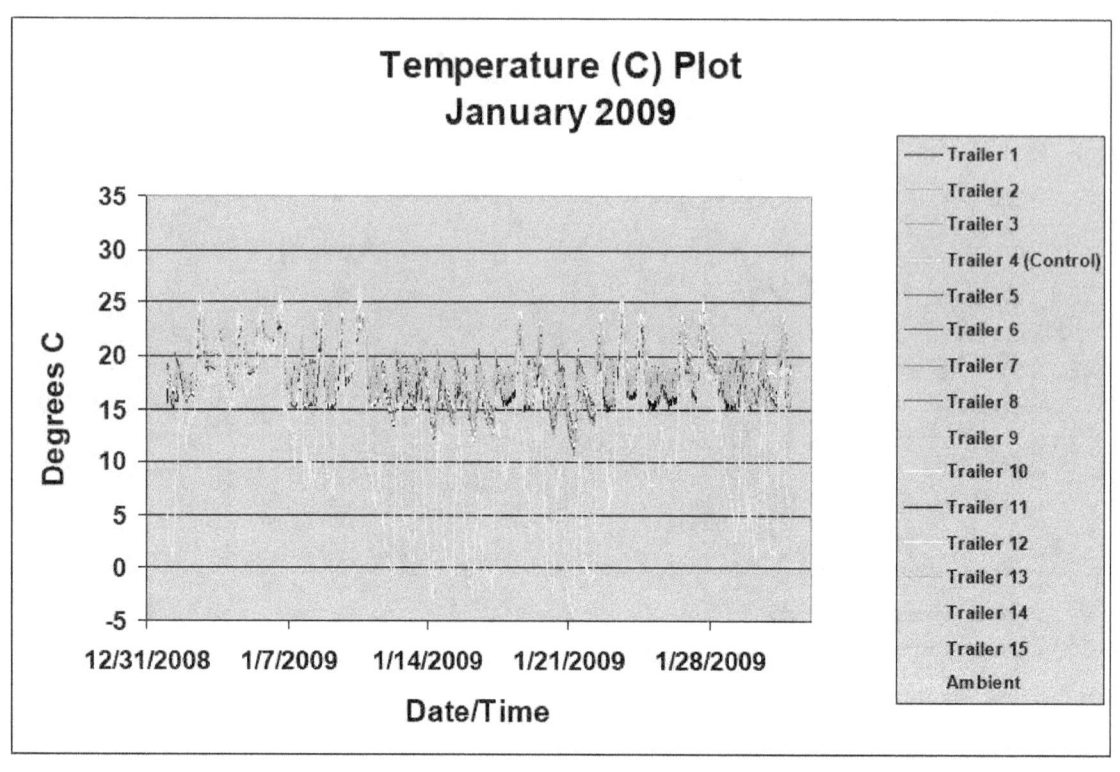

Temperature (C) Plot
January 2009

Legend: Trailer 1, Trailer 2, Trailer 3, Trailer 4 (Control), Trailer 5, Trailer 6, Trailer 7, Trailer 8, Trailer 9, Trailer 10, Trailer 11, Trailer 12, Trailer 13, Trailer 14, Trailer 15, Ambient

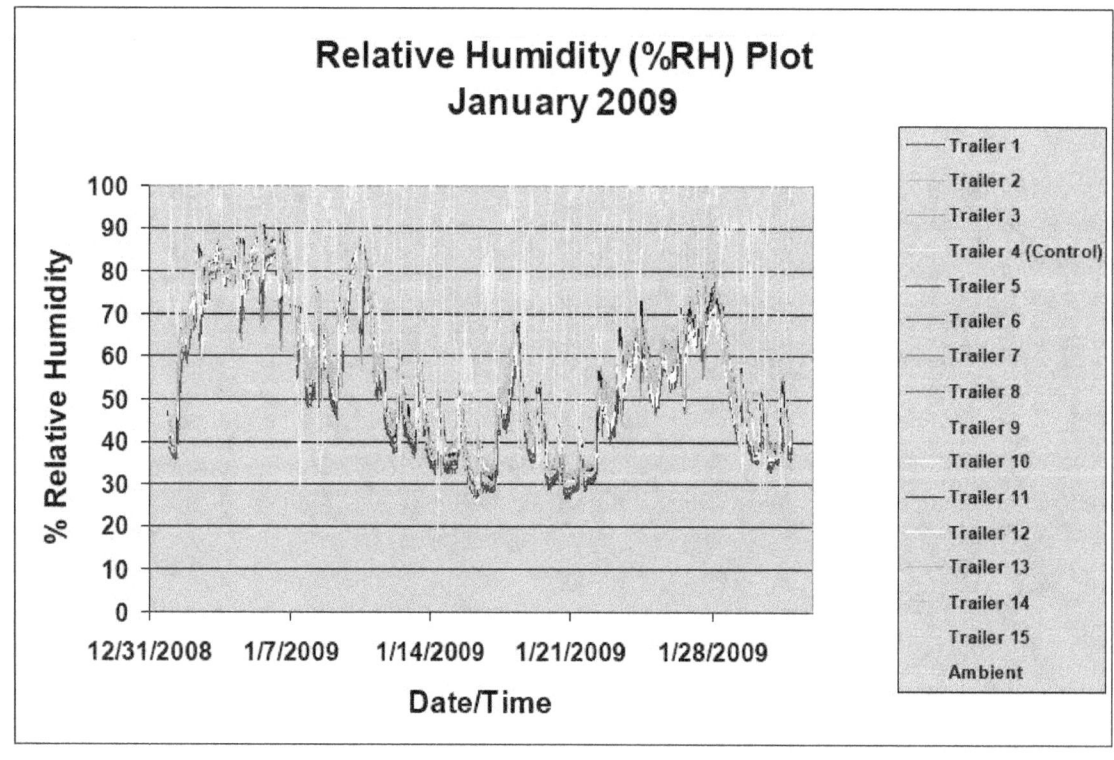

Relative Humidity (%RH) Plot
January 2009

Legend: Trailer 1, Trailer 2, Trailer 3, Trailer 4 (Control), Trailer 5, Trailer 6, Trailer 7, Trailer 8, Trailer 9, Trailer 10, Trailer 11, Trailer 12, Trailer 13, Trailer 14, Trailer 15, Ambient

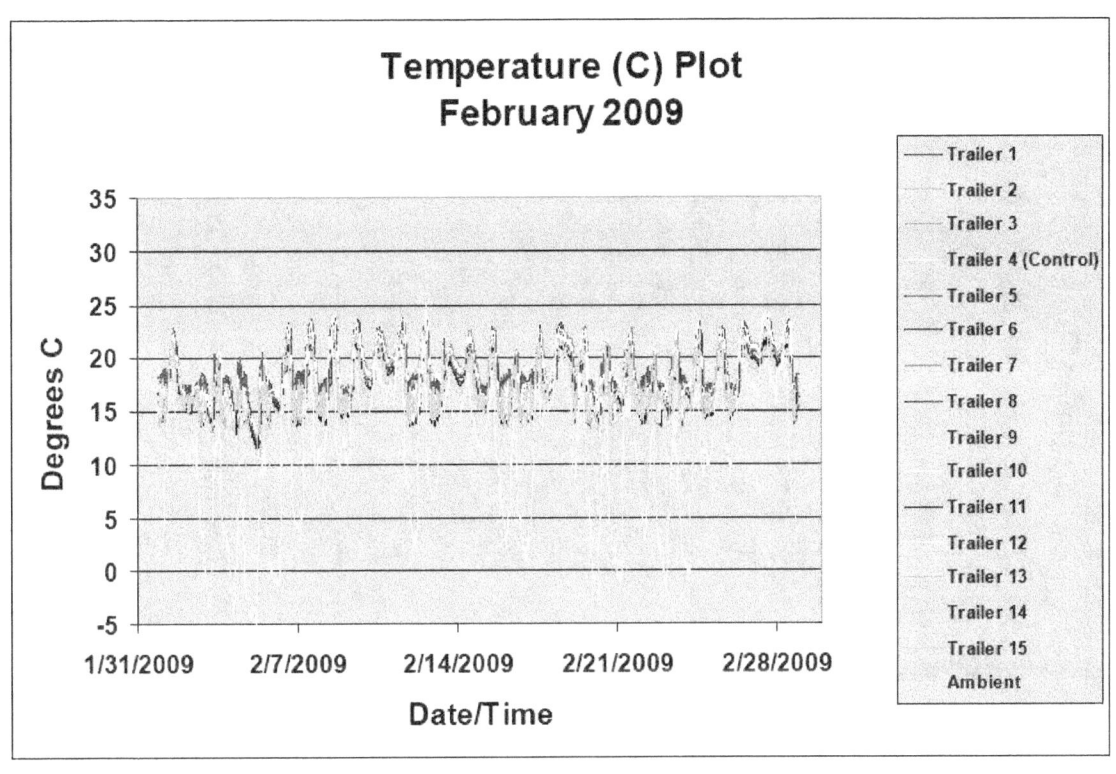

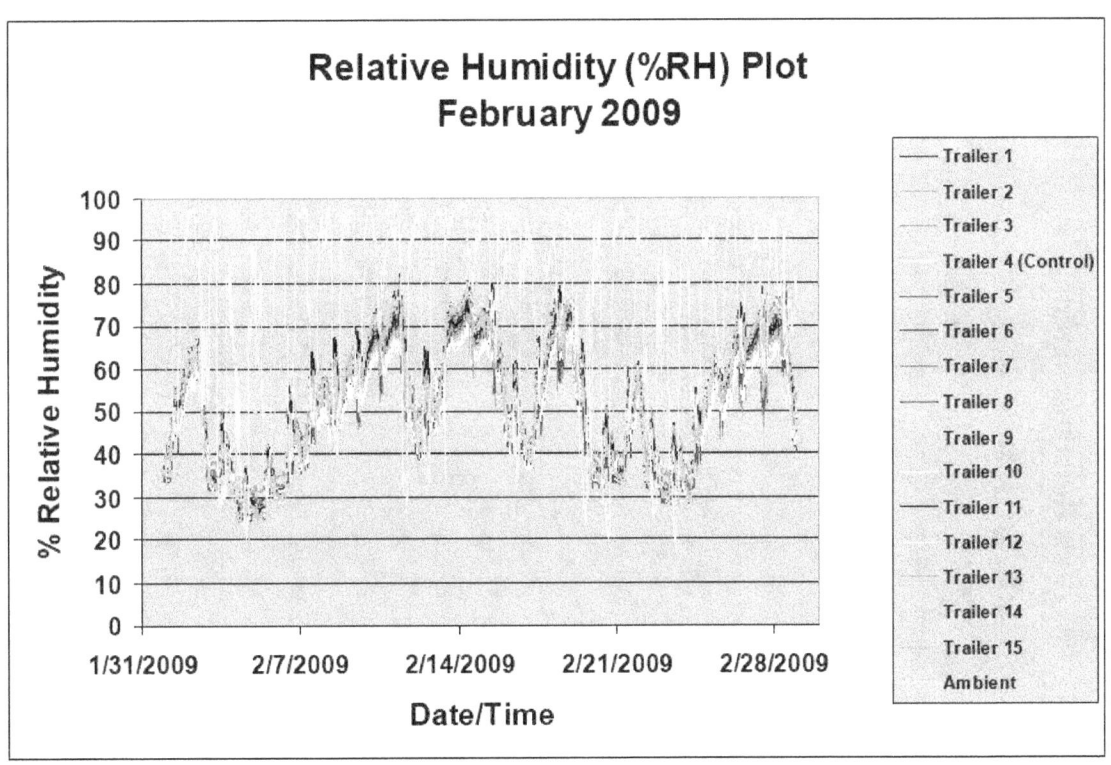

99

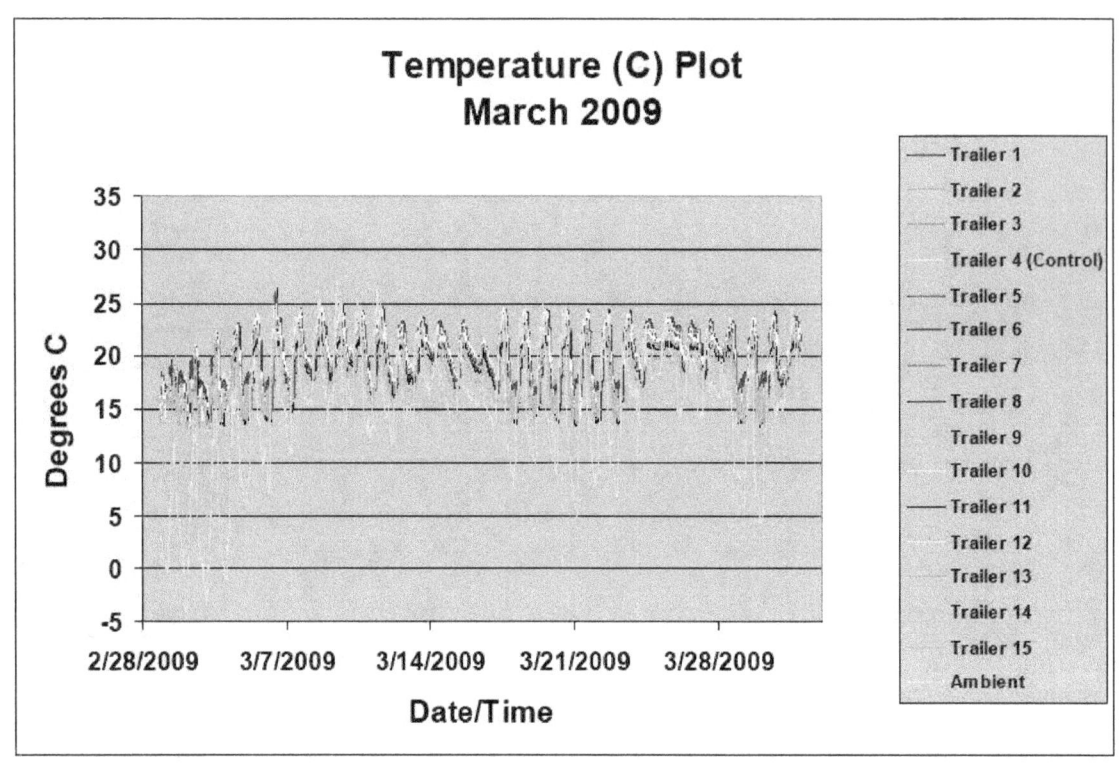

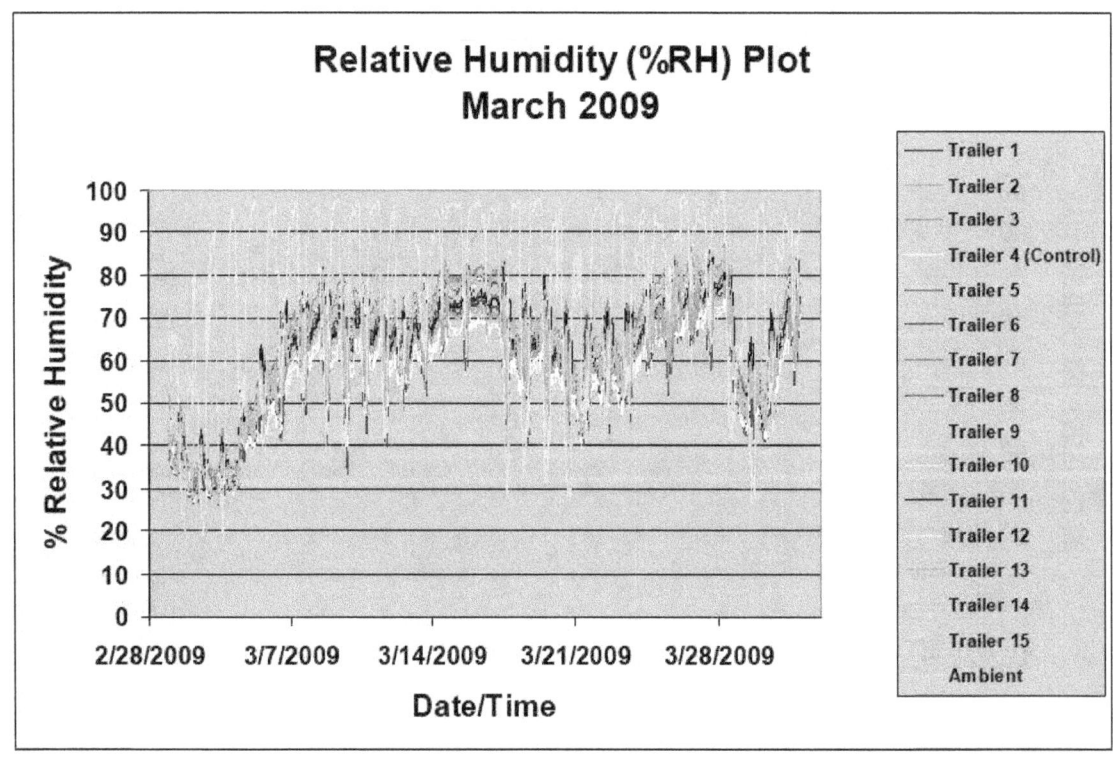

100

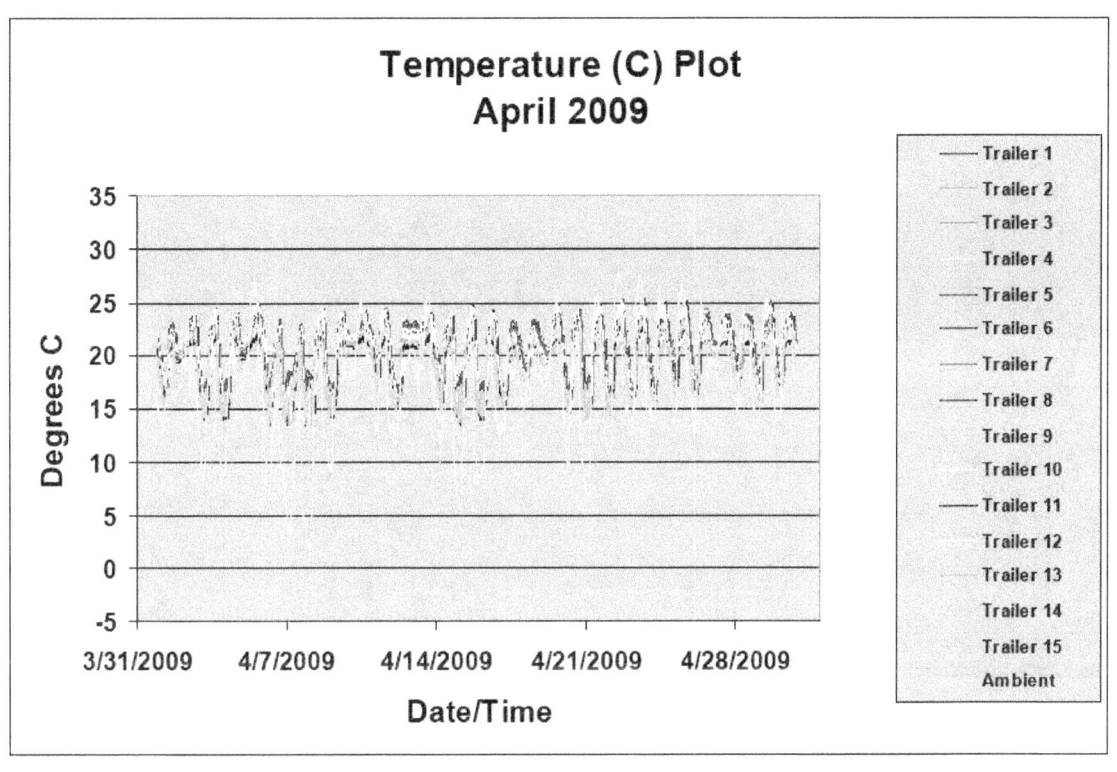

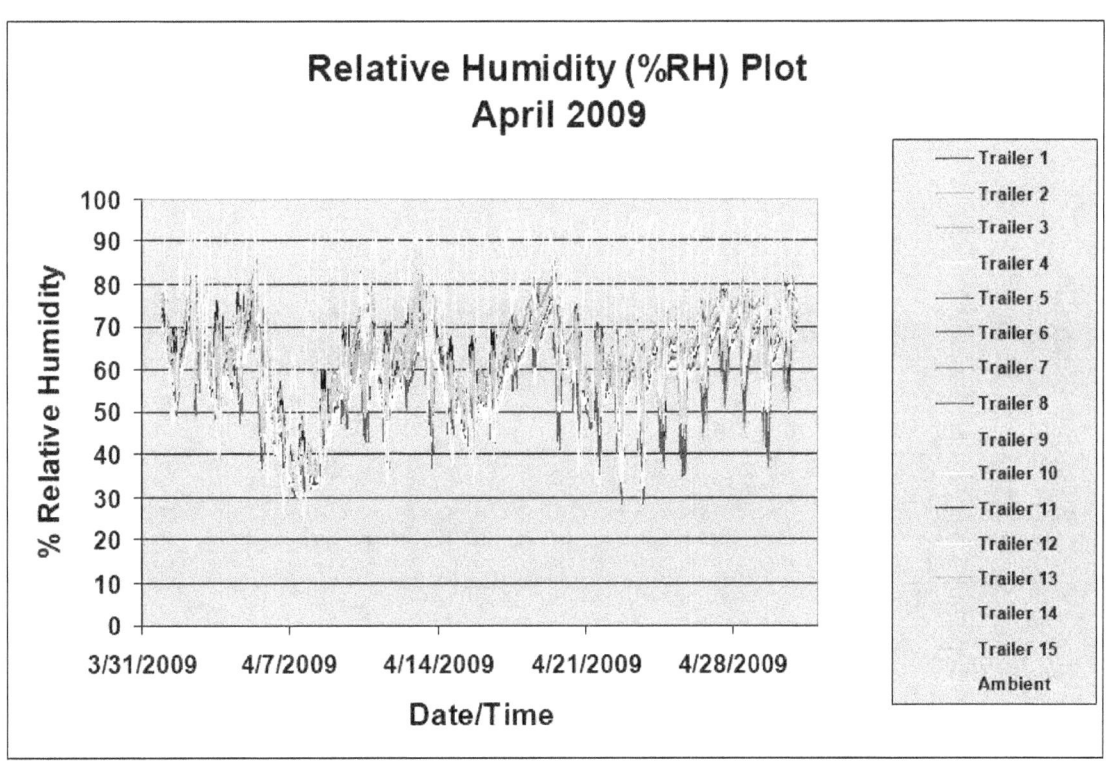

101

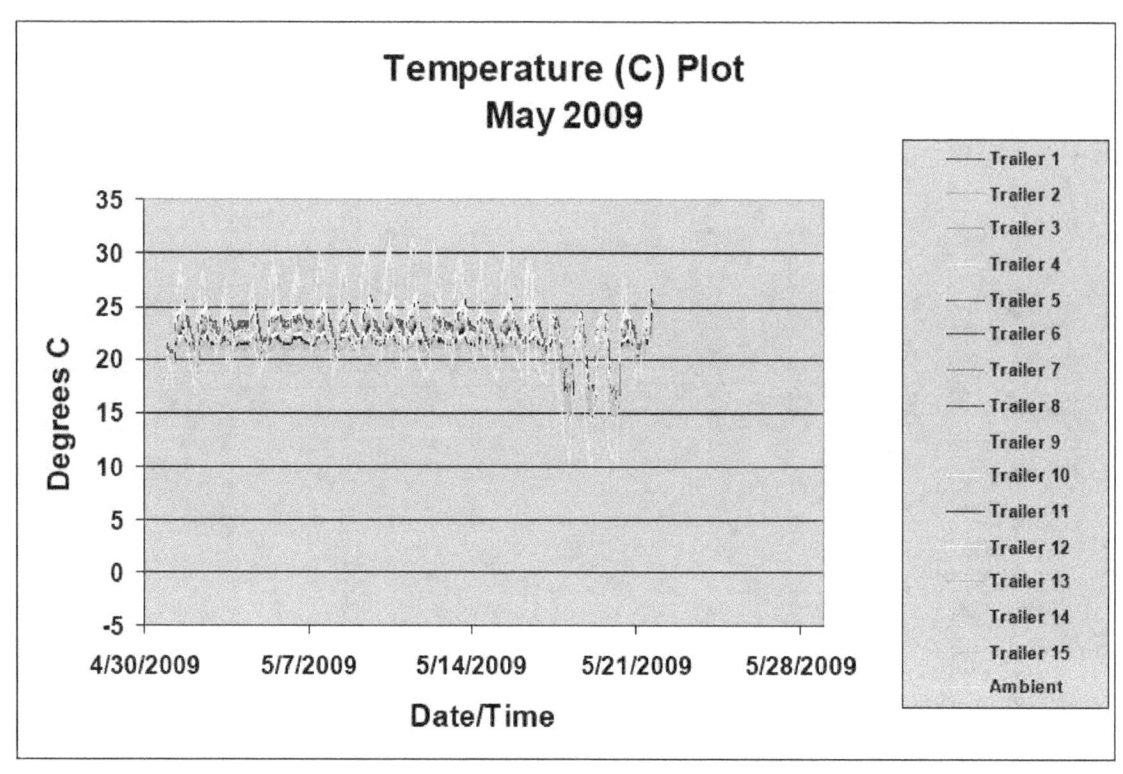

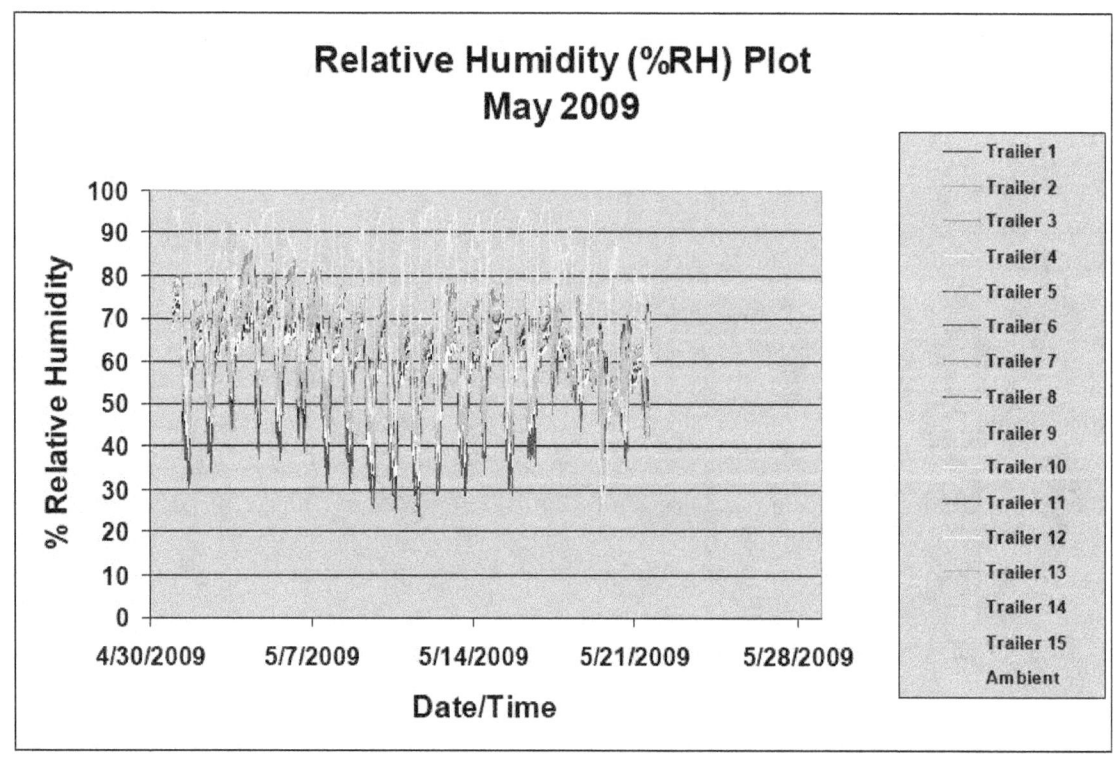

102

APPENDIX F

INDIVIDUAL AIR SAMPLING RESULTS

Formaldehyde, acetaldehyde, acetic acid, and TMPD-DIB air sample results. Trailer 16 is an ambient sample, 17 is a field blank, 18 is a media blank. NA–Not applicable. ND–Non-detected.

Date	Trailer	Analyte	Sample Duration (minutes)	Sample Volume (liters)	Sample Mass (µg)	Concentration (ppb)
12/16/2008	1	Acetic Acid	62	60.60	67	450
12/16/2008	2	Acetic Acid	60	47.80	38	320
12/16/2008	3	Acetic Acid	62	58.10	30	210
12/16/2008	4	Acetic Acid	60	49.00	32	270
12/16/2008	5	Acetic Acid	63	61.60	28	190
12/16/2008	6	Acetic Acid	62	61.80	25	170
12/16/2008	7	Acetic Acid	61	57.80	20	140
12/16/2008	8	Acetic Acid	61	58.70	56	390
12/16/2008	9	Acetic Acid	61	60.10	45	310
12/16/2008	10	Acetic Acid	60	49.30	6.0	50
12/16/2008	11	Acetic Acid	60	46.60	54	470
12/16/2008	12	Acetic Acid	67	66.40	38	230
12/16/2008	13	Acetic Acid	67	63.80	37	240
12/16/2008	14	Acetic Acid	81	81.90	22	110
12/16/2008	15	Acetic Acid	68	66.70	50	310
12/16/2008	16	Acetic Acid	60	46.60	ND	ND
12/16/2008	17	Acetic Acid	NA	NA	ND	ND
12/17/2008	1	Formaldehyde	64	31.70	21	540
12/17/2008	1	TMPD-DIB	64	13.00	ND	ND
12/17/2008	2	Formaldehyde	47	23.50	5.8	200
12/17/2008	2	TMPD-DIB	63	12.70	ND	ND
12/17/2008	3	Formaldehyde	14	6.96	2.0	230
12/17/2008	3	TMPD-DIB	64	12.90	ND	ND
12/17/2008	4	Formaldehyde	62	30.70	7.5	200
12/17/2008	4	TMPD-DIB	62	12.60	ND	ND
12/17/2008	5	Formaldehyde	60	29.80	7.0	190
12/17/2008	5	TMPD-DIB	60	12.10	ND	ND
12/17/2008	6	Formaldehyde	60	29.90	11	300
12/17/2008	6	TMPD-DIB	60	12.20	ND	ND
12/17/2008	7	Formaldehyde	60	30.30	9.5	260
12/17/2008	7	TMPD-DIB	60	12.10	ND	ND
12/17/2008	8	Formaldehyde	60	29.80	16	440
12/17/2008	8	TMPD-DIB	61	12.40	ND	ND
12/17/2008	9	Formaldehyde	60	30.20	13	350
12/17/2008	9	TMPD-DIB	60	12.20	ND	ND
12/17/2008	10	Formaldehyde	60	30.50	17	460
12/17/2008	10	TMPD-DIB	61	12.40	ND	ND
12/17/2008	11	Formaldehyde	60	29.60	17	470
12/17/2008	11	TMPD-DIB	59	11.90	ND	ND
12/17/2008	12	Formaldehyde	61	31.20	9.4	250
12/17/2008	12	TMPD-DIB	60	12.10	ND	ND
12/17/2008	13	Formaldehyde	60	30.00	9.3	250

104

Date	Trailer	Analyte	Sample Duration (minutes)	Sample Volume (liters)	Sample Mass (µg)	Concentration (ppb)
12/17/2008	13	TMPD-DIB	61	12.30	ND	ND
12/17/2008	14	Formaldehyde	60	31.40	7.5	200
12/17/2008	14	TMPD-DIB	60	12.10	ND	ND
12/17/2008	15	Formaldehyde	60	30.40	10	270
12/17/2008	15	TMPD-DIB	60	12.10	ND	ND
12/17/2008	16	Formaldehyde	63	31.60	ND	ND
12/17/2008	16	TMPD-DIB	64	13.00	ND	ND
12/17/2008	17	Formaldehyde	NA	NA	ND	ND
12/17/2008	17	TMPD-DIB	NA	NA	ND	ND
12/18/2008	1	Acetic Acid	63	52.20	25	200
12/18/2008	1	Formaldehyde	16	8.16	6.8	680
12/18/2008	2	Acetic Acid	65	52.00	19	150
12/18/2008	2	Formaldehyde	13	6.54	2.2	270
12/18/2008	3	Acetic Acid	65	50.50	11	89
12/18/2008	3	Formaldehyde	6	3.05	1.0	270
12/18/2008	4	Acetic Acid	65	52.50	21	160
12/18/2008	4	Formaldehyde	38	19.10	6.2	260
12/18/2008	5	Acetic Acid	65	51.90	21	170
12/18/2008	5	Formaldehyde	56	28.10	13	380
12/18/2008	6	Acetic Acid	67	54.30	14	110
12/18/2008	6	Formaldehyde	65	32.80	15	370
12/18/2008	7	Acetic Acid	68	54.80	15	110
12/18/2008	7	Formaldehyde	67	34.00	13	310
12/18/2008	8	Acetic Acid	68	54.80	22	160
12/18/2008	8	Formaldehyde	68	34.50	23	540
12/18/2008	9	Acetic Acid	68	56.80	20	140
12/18/2008	9	Formaldehyde	47	24.00	12	410
12/18/2008	10	Acetic Acid	68	57.60	46	330
12/18/2008	10	Formaldehyde	69	35.10	25	580
12/18/2008	11	Acetic Acid	69	56.30	43	310
12/18/2008	11	Formaldehyde	69	36.20	29	650
12/18/2008	12	Acetic Acid	69	57.60	21	150
12/18/2008	12	Formaldehyde	69	34.90	16	370
12/18/2008	13	Acetic Acid	68	57.50	20	140
12/18/2008	13	Formaldehyde	69	34.90	17	400
12/18/2008	14	Acetic Acid	69	54.70	16	120
12/18/2008	14	Formaldehyde	68	34.60	10	240
12/18/2008	15	Acetic Acid	70	57.60	18	130
12/18/2008	15	Formaldehyde	69	35.30	13	300
12/18/2008	16	Acetic Acid	71	59.10	ND	ND
12/18/2008	16	Formaldehyde	72	36.70	ND	ND
12/18/2008	17	Acetic Acid	NA	NA	ND	ND
12/18/2008	17	Formaldehyde	NA	NA	ND	ND
12/19/2008	1	TMPD-DIB	66	13.30	ND	ND

Date	Trailer	Analyte	Sample Duration (minutes)	Sample Volume (liters)	Sample Mass (μg)	Concentration (ppb)
12/19/2008	2	TMPD-DIB	69	14.00	ND	ND
12/19/2008	3	TMPD-DIB	70	14.30	ND	ND
12/19/2008	4	TMPD-DIB	71	14.40	ND	ND
12/19/2008	5	TMPD-DIB	70	14.30	ND	ND
12/19/2008	6	TMPD-DIB	71	14.50	ND	ND
12/19/2008	7	TMPD-DIB	72	14.60	ND	ND
12/19/2008	8	TMPD-DIB	64	13.10	ND	ND
12/19/2008	9	TMPD-DIB	63	12.80	ND	ND
12/19/2008	10	TMPD-DIB	61	12.40	ND	ND
12/19/2008	11	TMPD-DIB	60	12.10	ND	ND
12/19/2008	12	TMPD-DIB	60	12.20	ND	ND
12/19/2008	13	TMPD-DIB	60	12.20	ND	ND
12/19/2008	14	TMPD-DIB	60	12.20	ND	ND
12/19/2008	15	TMPD-DIB	60	12.30	ND	ND
12/19/2008	16	TMPD-DIB	60	12.20	ND	ND
12/19/2008	17	TMPD-DIB	NA	NA	ND	ND
1/13/2009	1	Acetic Acid	60	24.70	12	200
1/13/2009	1	Formaldehyde	60	29.90	9.5	260
1/13/2009	2	Acetic Acid	60	25.10	8.2	130
1/13/2009	2	Formaldehyde	60	30.00	3.3	90
1/13/2009	3	Acetic Acid	60	25.30	6.2	100
1/13/2009	3	Formaldehyde	60	32.30	4.3	110
1/13/2009	4	Acetic Acid	61	25.60	10	160
1/13/2009	4	Formaldehyde	60	30.20	4.4	120
1/13/2009	5	Acetic Acid	60	25.30	11	180
1/13/2009	5	Formaldehyde	60	30.60	5.5	150
1/13/2009	6	Acetic Acid	60	25.50	6.5	100
1/13/2009	6	Formaldehyde	60	30.00	4.7	130
1/13/2009	7	Acetic Acid	60	24.80	6.2	100
1/13/2009	7	Formaldehyde	60	30.90	3.6	95
1/13/2009	8	Acetic Acid	60	25.90	10	160
1/13/2009	8	Formaldehyde	60	30.20	7.6	210
1/13/2009	9	Acetic Acid	60	25.90	7.3	120
1/13/2009	9	Formaldehyde	60	29.90	6.0	160
1/13/2009	10	Acetic Acid	60	25.80	12	190
1/13/2009	10	Formaldehyde	60	30.00	8.9	240
1/13/2009	11	Acetic Acid	60	25.30	16	260
1/13/2009	11	Formaldehyde	60	30.30	12	320
1/13/2009	12	Acetic Acid	60	26.10	8.4	130
1/13/2009	12	Formaldehyde	60	30.30	5.4	150
1/13/2009	13	Acetic Acid	60	25.70	5.5	87
1/13/2009	13	Formaldehyde	60	30.20	6.0	160
1/13/2009	14	Acetic Acid	60	25.80	5.9	93
1/13/2009	14	Formaldehyde	60	30.40	3.6	96

Date	Trailer	Analyte	Sample Duration (minutes)	Sample Volume (liters)	Sample Mass (µg)	Concentration (ppb)
1/13/2009	15	Acetic Acid	60	25.60	10	160
1/13/2009	15	Formaldehyde	60	30.90	6.7	180
1/13/2009	16	Acetic Acid	60	25.70	ND	ND
1/13/2009	16	Formaldehyde	61	31.40	ND	ND
1/13/2009	17	Acetic Acid	NA	NA	ND	ND
1/13/2009	17	Formaldehyde	NA	NA	ND	ND
1/13/2009	18	Acetic Acid	0	NA	ND	ND
1/13/2009	18	Formaldehyde	0	NA	ND	ND
1/14/2009	1	Formaldehyde	60	30.10	6.9	190
1/14/2009	1	TMPD-DIB	60	12.20	ND	ND
1/14/2009	2	Formaldehyde	60	29.90	2.7	74
1/14/2009	2	TMPD-DIB	60	12.10	ND	ND
1/14/2009	3	Formaldehyde	60	30.20	2.4	65
1/14/2009	3	TMPD-DIB	60	12.20	ND	ND
1/14/2009	4	Formaldehyde	60	31.00	2.9	76
1/14/2009	4	TMPD-DIB	60	12.10	ND	ND
1/14/2009	5	Formaldehyde	60	30.70	4.4	120
1/14/2009	5	TMPD-DIB	60	12.10	ND	ND
1/14/2009	6	Formaldehyde	60	31.10	4.1	110
1/14/2009	6	TMPD-DIB	60	12.10	ND	ND
1/14/2009	7	Formaldehyde	60	30.80	2.6	69
1/14/2009	7	TMPD-DIB	60	12.20	ND	ND
1/14/2009	8	Formaldehyde	60	31.70	6.2	160
1/14/2009	8	TMPD-DIB	60	12.10	ND	ND
1/14/2009	9	Formaldehyde	60	30.00	4.8	130
1/14/2009	9	TMPD-DIB	60	12.10	ND	ND
1/14/2009	10	Formaldehyde	60	30.50	6.3	170
1/14/2009	10	TMPD-DIB	60	12.20	ND	ND
1/14/2009	11	Formaldehyde	60	31.20	7.5	200
1/14/2009	11	TMPD-DIB	60	12.10	ND	ND
1/14/2009	12	Formaldehyde	60	30.20	4.5	120
1/14/2009	12	TMPD-DIB	60	12.10	ND	ND
1/14/2009	13	Formaldehyde	60	30.30	6.6	180
1/14/2009	13	TMPD-DIB	60	12.10	ND	ND
1/14/2009	14	Formaldehyde	60	30.10	2.0	54
1/14/2009	14	TMPD-DIB	60	12.10	ND	ND
1/14/2009	15	Formaldehyde	60	30.80	4.0	110
1/14/2009	15	TMPD-DIB	60	12.10	ND	ND
1/14/2009	16	Formaldehyde	60	29.20	ND	ND
1/14/2009	16	TMPD-DIB	60	12.10	ND	ND
1/14/2009	17	Formaldehyde	NA	NA	ND	ND
1/14/2009	17	TMPD-DIB	NA	NA	ND	ND
1/15/2009	1	Acetic Acid	60	23.60	10	170
1/15/2009	1	Formaldehyde	60	30.70	7.6	200

Date	Trailer	Analyte	Sample Duration (minutes)	Sample Volume (liters)	Sample Mass (µg)	Concentration (ppb)
1/15/2009	2	Acetic Acid	61	24.00	7.5	130
1/15/2009	2	Formaldehyde	61	30.40	2.6	70
1/15/2009	3	Acetic Acid	61	24.10	4.6	78
1/15/2009	3	Formaldehyde	61	31.20	3.3	86
1/15/2009	4	Acetic Acid	60	23.60	8.9	150
1/15/2009	4	Formaldehyde	60	30.00	2.9	79
1/15/2009	5	Acetic Acid	60	23.90	8.4	140
1/15/2009	5	Formaldehyde	60	30.20	4.6	120
1/15/2009	6	Acetic Acid	60	23.70	7.5	130
1/15/2009	6	Formaldehyde	60	31.00	4.3	110
1/15/2009	7	Acetic Acid	62	24.40	6.6	110
1/15/2009	7	Formaldehyde	61	30.60	3.6	96
1/15/2009	8	Acetic Acid	60	23.90	9.1	160
1/15/2009	8	Formaldehyde	60	31.50	7.0	180
1/15/2009	9	Acetic Acid	60	23.90	7.4	130
1/15/2009	9	Formaldehyde	60	30.10	4.8	130
1/15/2009	10	Acetic Acid	60	23.60	12	210
1/15/2009	10	Formaldehyde	60	30.60	7.4	200
1/15/2009	11	Acetic Acid	60	23.80	13	220
1/15/2009	11	Formaldehyde	60	32.50	10	250
1/15/2009	12	Acetic Acid	60	23.60	6.0	100
1/15/2009	12	Formaldehyde	60	30.50	4.5	120
1/15/2009	13	Acetic Acid	60	23.80	5.4	92
1/15/2009	13	Formaldehyde	60	30.60	4.0	110
1/15/2009	14	Acetic Acid	60	23.90	5.4	92
1/15/2009	14	Formaldehyde	60	30.90	2.5	66
1/15/2009	15	Acetic Acid	61	24.30	6.3	110
1/15/2009	15	Formaldehyde	61	30.50	5.3	140
1/15/2009	16	Acetic Acid	61	24.00	ND	ND
1/15/2009	16	Formaldehyde	61	31.00	ND	ND
1/15/2009	17	Acetic Acid	NA	NA	ND	ND
1/15/2009	17	Formaldehyde	NA	NA	ND	ND
1/16/2009	1	Formaldehyde	60	30.10	5.8	160
1/16/2009	2	Formaldehyde	60	29.80	2.2	60
1/16/2009	3	Formaldehyde	60	29.70	2.2	60
1/16/2009	4	Formaldehyde	60	29.80	2.4	66
1/16/2009	5	Formaldehyde	60	29.90	3.7	100
1/16/2009	6	Formaldehyde	60	29.90	3.2	87
1/16/2009	7	Formaldehyde	60	30.10	3.3	89
1/16/2009	8	Formaldehyde	60	30.20	5.8	160
1/16/2009	9	Formaldehyde	60	29.60	3.6	99
1/16/2009	10	Formaldehyde	60	30.90	6.1	160
1/16/2009	11	Formaldehyde	60	29.90	6.1	170
1/16/2009	12	Formaldehyde	60	30.10	3.4	92

Date	Trailer	Analyte	Sample Duration (minutes)	Sample Volume (liters)	Sample Mass (μg)	Concentration (ppb)
1/16/2009	13	Formaldehyde	60	29.90		Pump Fail
1/16/2009	14	Formaldehyde	60	30.60	2.0	53
1/16/2009	15	Formaldehyde	60	29.70	3.7	100
1/16/2009	16	Formaldehyde	60	29.70	ND	ND
1/16/2009	17	Formaldehyde	NA	NA	ND	ND
1/17/2009	1	Formaldehyde	60	31.00	5.7	150
1/17/2009	2	Formaldehyde	60	30.80	2.0	53
1/17/2009	3	Formaldehyde	60	30.00	2.0	54
1/17/2009	4	Formaldehyde	60	30.00	2.3	62
1/17/2009	5	Formaldehyde	60	32.20	5.3	130
1/17/2009	6	Formaldehyde	60	30.30	3.1	83
1/17/2009	7	Formaldehyde	60	30.50	1.9	51
1/17/2009	8	Formaldehyde	60	30.10	4.4	120
1/17/2009	9	Formaldehyde	60	31.80	3.3	84
1/17/2009	10	Formaldehyde	60	31.10	6.1	160
1/17/2009	11	Formaldehyde	60	30.10	3.4	92
1/17/2009	12	Formaldehyde	60	31.20	3.4	89
1/17/2009	13	Formaldehyde	60	30.80	3.6	95
1/17/2009	14	Formaldehyde	60	30.20	2.1	57
1/17/2009	15	Formaldehyde	60	30.80	4.6	120
1/17/2009	16	Formaldehyde	60	30.30	ND	ND
1/17/2009	17	Formaldehyde	NA	NA	ND	ND
1/18/2009	1	Acetaldehyde	65	33.40	0.30	5.0
1/18/2009	1	Formaldehyde	65	33.40	11	270
1/18/2009	2	Formaldehyde	66	33.60	5.2	130
1/18/2009	3	Formaldehyde	64	33.00	6.7	170
1/18/2009	4	Formaldehyde	61	30.80	5.8	150
1/18/2009	5	Formaldehyde	62	32.20	7.2	180
1/18/2009	6	Acetaldehyde	63	33.30	0.30	5.0
1/18/2009	6	Formaldehyde	63	33.30	8.6	210
1/18/2009	7	Formaldehyde	66	33.70	7.2	170
1/18/2009	8	Formaldehyde	63	31.80	3.6	92
1/18/2009	9	Formaldehyde	63	34.10	3.0	72
1/18/2009	10	Acetaldehyde	60	30.50	0.70	13
1/18/2009	10	Formaldehyde	60	30.50	7.9	210
1/18/2009	11	Acetaldehyde	67	34.20	0.60	9.7
1/18/2009	11	Formaldehyde	67	34.20	16	380
1/18/2009	12	Acetaldehyde	63	32.50	0.30	5.1
1/18/2009	12	Formaldehyde	63	32.50	5.1	130
1/18/2009	13	Acetaldehyde	61	31.50	0.60	11
1/18/2009	13	Formaldehyde	61	31.50	4.6	120
1/18/2009	14	Formaldehyde	64	32.70	4.4	110
1/18/2009	15	Formaldehyde	63	32.70	7.3	180
1/18/2009	16	Formaldehyde	60	30.90	ND	ND

Date	Trailer	Analyte	Sample Duration (minutes)	Sample Volume (liters)	Sample Mass (µg)	Concentration (ppb)
1/18/2009	17	Formaldehyde	NA	NA	ND	ND
1/19/2009	1	Formaldehyde	60	30.90	9.2	240
1/19/2009	2	Formaldehyde	60	30.60	3.7	99
1/19/2009	3	Formaldehyde	60	31.40	4.0	100
1/19/2009	4	Formaldehyde	60	31.40	4.1	110
1/19/2009	5	Formaldehyde	60	31.00	5.0	130
1/19/2009	6	Formaldehyde	60	30.20	5.0	140
1/19/2009	7	Formaldehyde	60	31.20	5.1	130
1/19/2009	8	Formaldehyde	60	31.10	2.3	60
1/19/2009	9	Formaldehyde	60	30.20	1.7	46
1/19/2009	10	Acetaldehyde	60	30.20	0.40	7.4
1/19/2009	10	Formaldehyde	60	30.20	4.8	130
1/19/2009	11	Acetaldehyde	60	30.10	0.50	9.2
1/19/2009	11	Formaldehyde	60	30.10	12	320
1/19/2009	12	Acetaldehyde	60	30.30	0.20	3.7
1/19/2009	12	Formaldehyde	60	30.30	2.8	75
1/19/2009	13	Acetaldehyde	60	30.10	0.30	5.5
1/19/2009	13	Formaldehyde	60	30.10	3.1	84
1/19/2009	14	Formaldehyde	60	30.60	2.7	72
1/19/2009	15	Formaldehyde	60	30.10	4.4	120
1/19/2009	16	Formaldehyde	60	30.00	ND	ND
1/19/2009	17	Formaldehyde	NA	NA	ND	ND
1/20/2009	1	Acetic Acid	61	23.60	6.0	100
1/20/2009	1	Formaldehyde	61	30.60	4.2	110
1/20/2009	2	Acetic Acid	61	23.60	6.0	100
1/20/2009	2	Formaldehyde	61	30.10	2.0	54
1/20/2009	3	Acetic Acid	61	23.80	3.0	51
1/20/2009	3	Formaldehyde	61	30.50	1.6	43
1/20/2009	4	Acetic Acid	60	23.50	6.0	100
1/20/2009	4	Formaldehyde	60	30.00	1.6	43
1/20/2009	5	Acetic Acid	60	23.70	4.0	69
1/20/2009	5	Formaldehyde	60	29.80	1.6	44
1/20/2009	6	Acetic Acid	60	23.40	3.0	52
1/20/2009	6	Formaldehyde	60	29.80	2.1	57
1/20/2009	7	Acetic Acid	60	23.20	4.0	70
1/20/2009	7	Formaldehyde	60	30.30	2.3	62
1/20/2009	8	Acetic Acid	60	23.60	6.0	100
1/20/2009	8	Formaldehyde	60	29.60	0.70	19
1/20/2009	9	Acetic Acid	60	23.40	3.0	52
1/20/2009	9	Formaldehyde	60	30.00	0.40	11
1/20/2009	10	Acetic Acid	60	23.60	5.0	86
1/20/2009	10	Formaldehyde	60	29.90	2.0	55
1/20/2009	11	Acetic Acid	60	23.60	9.0	160
1/20/2009	11	Formaldehyde	60	30.80	3.2	85

Date	Trailer	Analyte	Sample Duration (minutes)	Sample Volume (liters)	Sample Mass (μg)	Concentration (ppb)
1/20/2009	12	Acetic Acid	60	23.60	4.0	69
1/20/2009	12	Formaldehyde	60	29.90	0.9	25
1/20/2009	13	Acetic Acid	60	23.10	4.0	71
1/20/2009	13	Formaldehyde	60	29.80	1.0	27
1/20/2009	14	Acetic Acid	60	23.50	3.0	52
1/20/2009	14	Formaldehyde	60	29.90	1.2	33
1/20/2009	15	Acetic Acid	61	24.30	2.0	34
1/20/2009	15	Formaldehyde	61	31.40	1.9	49
1/20/2009	16	Acetic Acid	61	24.30	ND	ND
1/20/2009	16	Formaldehyde	61	31.40	ND	ND
1/20/2009	17	Acetic Acid	NA	NA	ND	ND
1/20/2009	17	Formaldehyde	NA	NA	ND	ND
1/21/2009	1	Formaldehyde	60	30.30	6.4	170
1/21/2009	1	TMPD-DIB	60	12.00	ND	ND
1/21/2009	2	Formaldehyde	60	30.10	2.4	65
1/21/2009	2	TMPD-DIB	60	12.00	ND	ND
1/21/2009	3	Formaldehyde	60	29.90	2.8	76
1/21/2009	3	TMPD-DIB	60	12.00	ND	ND
1/21/2009	4	Formaldehyde	60	30.10	2.8	76
1/21/2009	4	TMPD-DIB	60	12.00	ND	ND
1/21/2009	5	Formaldehyde	60	29.50	3.3	91
1/21/2009	5	TMPD-DIB	60	12.10	ND	ND
1/21/2009	6	Formaldehyde	60	30.10	3.4	92
1/21/2009	6	TMPD-DIB	60	12.00	ND	ND
1/21/2009	7	Formaldehyde	60	30.10	3.0	81
1/21/2009	7	TMPD-DIB	60	12.10	ND	ND
1/21/2009	8	Formaldehyde	60	29.90	1.7	46
1/21/2009	8	TMPD-DIB	60	12.10	ND	ND
1/21/2009	9	Formaldehyde	60	30.00	0.70	19
1/21/2009	9	TMPD-DIB	60	12.10	ND	ND
1/21/2009	10	Formaldehyde	60	30.00	2.9	79
1/21/2009	10	TMPD-DIB	60	12.10	ND	ND
1/21/2009	11	Formaldehyde	60	29.90	7.5	200
1/21/2009	11	TMPD-DIB	60	12.10	ND	ND
1/21/2009	12	Formaldehyde	60	30.60	1.9	51
1/21/2009	12	TMPD-DIB	60	12.10	ND	ND
1/21/2009	13	Formaldehyde	60	31.10	1.8	47
1/21/2009	13	TMPD-DIB	60	12.10	ND	ND
1/21/2009	14	Formaldehyde	60	30.40	2.0	54
1/21/2009	14	TMPD-DIB	60	12.10	ND	ND
1/21/2009	15	Formaldehyde	60	29.80	3.1	85
1/21/2009	15	TMPD-DIB	60	12.10	ND	ND
1/21/2009	16	Formaldehyde	60	31.10	ND	ND
1/21/2009	16	TMPD-DIB	60	12.10	ND	ND

Date	Trailer	Analyte	Sample Duration (minutes)	Sample Volume (liters)	Sample Mass (µg)	Concentration (ppb)
1/21/2009	17	Formaldehyde	NA	NA	ND	ND
1/21/2009	17	TMPD-DIB	NA	NA	ND	ND
1/22/2009	1	Formaldehyde	61	31.60	12	310
1/22/2009	2	Formaldehyde	60	30.70	4.8	130
1/22/2009	3	Formaldehyde	60	31.20	5.3	140
1/22/2009	4	Formaldehyde	60	31.40	6.0	160
1/22/2009	5	Formaldehyde	61	31.70	7.0	180
1/22/2009	6	Acetaldehyde	60	31.00	0.20	3.6
1/22/2009	6	Formaldehyde	60	31.00	7.4	190
1/22/2009	7	Formaldehyde	60	31.20	5.7	150
1/22/2009	8	Formaldehyde	61	31.80	3.3	84
1/22/2009	9	Formaldehyde	60	31.30	2.3	60
1/22/2009	10	Acetaldehyde	60	29.80	0.40	7.5
1/22/2009	10	Formaldehyde	60	29.80	6.2	170
1/22/2009	11	Acetaldehyde	60	30.20	0.40	7.3
1/22/2009	11	Formaldehyde	60	30.20	16	430
1/22/2009	12	Formaldehyde	60	31.20	4.1	110
1/22/2009	13	Acetaldehyde	60	30.00	0.40	7.4
1/22/2009	13	Formaldehyde	60	30.00	3.9	110
1/22/2009	14	Formaldehyde	61	30.30	4.4	120
1/22/2009	15	Formaldehyde	60	31.30	6.3	160
1/22/2009	16	Formaldehyde	61	30.60	ND	ND
1/22/2009	17	Formaldehyde	NA	NA	ND	ND
1/23/2009	1	Acetaldehyde	60	31.50	0.30	5.3
1/23/2009	1	Acetic Acid	60	24.20	15	250
1/23/2009	1	Formaldehyde	60	31.50	16	410
1/23/2009	2	Acetic Acid	60	24.50	12	200
1/23/2009	2	Formaldehyde	60	31.80	6.1	160
1/23/2009	3	Acetaldehyde	45	23.20	0.20	4.8
1/23/2009	3	Acetic Acid	60	24.10	4.4	74
1/23/2009	3	Formaldehyde	45	23.20	5.9	210
1/23/2009	4	Acetic Acid	61	24.90	12	200
1/23/2009	4	Formaldehyde	28	14.90	3.9	210
1/23/2009	5	Acetaldehyde	60	31.90	0.30	5.2
1/23/2009	5	Acetic Acid	60	24.10	13	220
1/23/2009	5	Formaldehyde	60	31.90	10	260
1/23/2009	6	Acetaldehyde	60	31.90	0.30	5.2
1/23/2009	6	Acetic Acid	60	24.30	9.6	160
1/23/2009	6	Formaldehyde	60	31.90	11	280
1/23/2009	7	Acetic Acid	60	24.20	8.5	140
1/23/2009	7	Formaldehyde	60	31.30	8.3	220
1/23/2009	8	Acetic Acid	60	24.10	6.2	110
1/23/2009	8	Formaldehyde	60	31.90	4.0	100
1/23/2009	9	Acetic Acid	60	24.50	4.0	67

Date	Trailer	Analyte	Sample Duration (minutes)	Sample Volume (liters)	Sample Mass (μg)	Concentration (ppb)
1/23/2009	9	Formaldehyde	60	31.10	3.1	81
1/23/2009	10	Acetaldehyde	60	31.90	0.80	14
1/23/2009	10	Acetic Acid	60	24.40	8.5	140
1/23/2009	10	Formaldehyde	60	31.90	9.5	240
1/23/2009	11	Acetaldehyde	60	31.40	0.60	11
1/23/2009	11	Acetic Acid	60	24.10	17	290
1/23/2009	11	Formaldehyde	60	31.40	21	540
1/23/2009	12	Acetaldehyde	60	32.10	0.30	5.2
1/23/2009	12	Acetic Acid	60	24.00	4.8	81
1/23/2009	12	Formaldehyde	60	32.10	5.4	140
1/23/2009	13	Acetaldehyde	60	32.70	0.70	12
1/23/2009	13	Acetic Acid	60	24.60	3.7	61
1/23/2009	13	Formaldehyde	60	32.70	6.0	150
1/23/2009	14	Acetaldehyde	60	31.90	0.20	3.5
1/23/2009	14	Acetic Acid	60	24.60	7.2	120
1/23/2009	14	Formaldehyde	60	31.90	5.8	150
1/23/2009	15	Acetic Acid	60	24.50	7.1	120
1/23/2009	15	Formaldehyde	60	31.80	7.4	190
1/23/2009	16	Acetic Acid	60	24.30	ND	ND
1/23/2009	16	Formaldehyde	60	30.90	ND	ND
1/23/2009	17	Acetic Acid	NA	NA	ND	ND
1/23/2009	17	Formaldehyde	NA	NA	ND	ND
1/24/2009	1	Acetaldehyde	62	31.10	0.30	5.3
1/24/2009	1	Formaldehyde	62	31.10	17	440
1/24/2009	2	Formaldehyde	60	30.50	7.2	190
1/24/2009	3	Formaldehyde	60	31.00	8.3	220
1/24/2009	4	Formaldehyde	0	30.90	8.1	210
1/24/2009	5	Formaldehyde	62	31.70	9.5	240
1/24/2009	6	Acetaldehyde	60	30.70	0.20	3.6
1/24/2009	6	Formaldehyde	60	30.70	9.8	260
1/24/2009	7	Formaldehyde	61	30.70	9.8	260
1/24/2009	8	Formaldehyde	61	30.70	3.9	100
1/24/2009	9	Formaldehyde	62	32.10	2.9	74
1/24/2009	10	Acetaldehyde	60	30.90	0.90	16
1/24/2009	10	Formaldehyde	60	30.90	9.6	250
1/24/2009	11	Acetaldehyde	62	31.80	0.40	7.0
1/24/2009	11	Formaldehyde	62	31.80	20	510
1/24/2009	12	Acetaldehyde	62	31.60	0.30	5.3
1/24/2009	12	Formaldehyde	62	31.60	4.9	130
1/24/2009	13	Acetaldehyde	60	30.90	0.70	13
1/24/2009	13	Formaldehyde	60	30.90	6.0	160
1/24/2009	14	Formaldehyde	62	31.50	5.5	140
1/24/2009	15	Formaldehyde	60	30.90	7.8	210
1/24/2009	16	Formaldehyde	62	31.50	ND	ND

Date	Trailer	Analyte	Sample Duration (minutes)	Sample Volume (liters)	Sample Mass (µg)	Concentration (ppb)
1/24/2009	17	Formaldehyde	NA	NA	ND	ND
1/25/2009	1	Formaldehyde	61	30.40	7.6	200
1/25/2009	2	Formaldehyde	61	30.40	3.1	83
1/25/2009	3	Formaldehyde	61	30.30	3.3	89
1/25/2009	4	Formaldehyde	62	31.00	3.4	90
1/25/2009	5	Formaldehyde	60	29.50	3.3	90
1/25/2009	6	Formaldehyde	61	30.60	4.1	110
1/25/2009	7	Formaldehyde	61	30.70	4.1	110
1/25/2009	8	Formaldehyde	61	30.00	1.6	44
1/25/2009	9	Formaldehyde	60	29.80	1	27
1/25/2009	10	Acetaldehyde	62	31.10	0.30	5.4
1/25/2009	10	Formaldehyde	62	31.10	3.4	89
1/25/2009	11	Acetaldehyde	61	30.70	0.20	3.6
1/25/2009	11	Formaldehyde	61	30.70	8.1	220
1/25/2009	12	Formaldehyde	61	30.60	2	53
1/25/2009	13	Acetaldehyde	61	30.40	0.20	3.6
1/25/2009	13	Formaldehyde	61	30.40	1.9	51
1/25/2009	14	Formaldehyde	62	31.30	2.2	57
1/25/2009	15	Formaldehyde	61	30.90	3.1	82
1/25/2009	16	Formaldehyde	61	30.70	ND	ND
1/25/2009	17	Formaldehyde	NA	NA	ND	ND
1/26/2009	1	Formaldehyde	60	31.70	17	440
1/26/2009	1	TMPD-DIB	60	12.10	ND	ND
1/26/2009	2	Formaldehyde	60	30.30	5.3	140
1/26/2009	2	TMPD-DIB	60	12.10	ND	ND
1/26/2009	3	Formaldehyde	60	30.30	6.5	170
1/26/2009	3	TMPD-DIB	60	12.10	ND	ND
1/26/2009	4	Formaldehyde	60	30.90	6.9	180
1/26/2009	4	TMPD-DIB	60	12.10	ND	ND
1/26/2009	5	Formaldehyde	60	30.70	8.3	220
1/26/2009	5	TMPD-DIB	60	12.10	ND	ND
1/26/2009	6	Formaldehyde	60	30.70	8.3	220
1/26/2009	6	TMPD-DIB	60	12.10	ND	ND
1/26/2009	7	Formaldehyde	60	31.20	6.6	170
1/26/2009	7	TMPD-DIB	60	12.20	ND	ND
1/26/2009	8	Formaldehyde	60	30.90	3.3	87
1/26/2009	8	TMPD-DIB	60	12.10	ND	ND
1/26/2009	9	Formaldehyde	60	30.40	1.9	51
1/26/2009	9	TMPD-DIB	60	12.20	ND	ND
1/26/2009	10	Acetaldehyde	60	30.40	0.60	11
1/26/2009	10	Formaldehyde	60	30.40	8.3	220
1/26/2009	10	TMPD-DIB	60	12.20	ND	ND
1/26/2009	11	Acetaldehyde	60	31.10	0.40	7.1
1/26/2009	11	Formaldehyde	60	31.10	19	500

Date	Trailer	Analyte	Sample Duration (minutes)	Sample Volume (liters)	Sample Mass (µg)	Concentration (ppb)
1/26/2009	11	TMPD-DIB	60	12.10	ND	ND
1/26/2009	12	Acetaldehyde	60	30.60	0.30	5.4
1/26/2009	12	Formaldehyde	60	30.60	4.4	120
1/26/2009	12	TMPD-DIB	60	12.10	ND	ND
1/26/2009	13	Acetaldehyde	60	30.70	0.50	9.0
1/26/2009	13	Formaldehyde	60	30.70	4.4	120
1/26/2009	13	TMPD-DIB	60	12.10	ND	ND
1/26/2009	14	Formaldehyde	60	30.50	4.8	130
1/26/2009	14	TMPD-DIB	60	12.20	ND	ND
1/26/2009	15	Formaldehyde	60	30.40	6.5	170
1/26/2009	15	TMPD-DIB	60	12.10	ND	ND
1/26/2009	16	Formaldehyde	60	30.20	ND	ND
1/26/2009	16	TMPD-DIB	60	12.10	ND	ND
1/26/2009	17	Formaldehyde	NA	NA	ND	ND
1/26/2009	17	TMPD-DIB	NA	NA	ND	ND
1/28/2009	1	Formaldehyde	66	32.70	9.2	230
1/28/2009	2	Formaldehyde	60	28.90	3.7	100
1/28/2009	3	Formaldehyde	60	29.60	4.7	130
1/28/2009	4	Formaldehyde	60	29.40	4.2	120
1/28/2009	5	Formaldehyde	60	29.40	4.1	110
1/28/2009	6	Formaldehyde	61	30.50	5.7	150
1/28/2009	7	Formaldehyde	64	31.90	5.1	130
1/28/2009	8	Formaldehyde	60	29.30	1.9	53
1/28/2009	9	Formaldehyde	65	31.70	1.6	41
1/28/2009	10	Acetaldehyde	65	31.60	0.60	11
1/28/2009	10	Formaldehyde	65	31.60	4.6	120
1/28/2009	11	Acetaldehyde	63	31.40	0.30	5.3
1/28/2009	11	Formaldehyde	63	31.40	12	310
1/28/2009	12	Acetaldehyde	66	32.60	0.30	5.1
1/28/2009	12	Formaldehyde	66	32.60	3.1	77
1/28/2009	13	Acetaldehyde	60	29.80	0.50	9.3
1/28/2009	13	Formaldehyde	60	29.80	3.2	88
1/28/2009	14	Formaldehyde	66	32.60	3.6	90
1/28/2009	15	Formaldehyde	60	29.70	4.4	120
1/28/2009	16	Formaldehyde	63	31.20	ND	ND
1/28/2009	17	Formaldehyde	NA	NA	ND	ND
1/30/2009	1	Acetic Acid	60	24.00	10	170
1/30/2009	1	Formaldehyde	60	29.60	7.6	210
1/30/2009	2	Acetic Acid	60	24.00	8.0	140
1/30/2009	2	Formaldehyde	60	29.80	3.2	87
1/30/2009	3	Acetic Acid	60	24.10	5.0	85
1/30/2009	3	Formaldehyde	60	30.00	2.9	79
1/30/2009	4	Acetic Acid	60	23.90	9.0	150
1/30/2009	4	Formaldehyde	60	29.80	3.5	96

115

Date	Trailer	Analyte	Sample Duration (minutes)	Sample Volume (liters)	Sample Mass (μg)	Concentration (ppb)
1/30/2009	5	Acetic Acid	60	23.90	10	170
1/30/2009	5	Formaldehyde	60	29.70	3.9	110
1/30/2009	6	Acetic Acid	60	23.60	8.0	140
1/30/2009	6	Formaldehyde	60	30.00	4.2	110
1/30/2009	7	Acetic Acid	60	24.10	7.0	120
1/30/2009	7	Formaldehyde	60	33.40	4.8	120
1/30/2009	8	Acetic Acid	60	24.10	9.0	150
1/30/2009	8	Formaldehyde	60	30.20	2.3	62
1/30/2009	9	Acetic Acid	60	23.70	4.0	69
1/30/2009	9	Formaldehyde	60	29.70	0.9	25
1/30/2009	10	Acetaldehyde	60	29.90	0.3	5.6
1/30/2009	10	Acetic Acid	60	23.90	7.0	120
1/30/2009	10	Formaldehyde	60	29.90	3.8	100
1/30/2009	11	Acetaldehyde	60	30.00	0.30	5.6
1/30/2009	11	Acetic Acid	60	23.90	16	270
1/30/2009	11	Formaldehyde	60	30.00	11	300
1/30/2009	12	Acetic Acid	60	23.90	5.0	85
1/30/2009	12	Formaldehyde	60	29.80	2.1	57
1/30/2009	13	Acetaldehyde	60	30.20	0.3	5.5
1/30/2009	13	Acetic Acid	60	23.80	5.0	85
1/30/2009	13	Formaldehyde	60	30.20	2.3	62
1/30/2009	14	Acetaldehyde	60	30.10	0.20	3.7
1/30/2009	14	Acetic Acid	60	24.10	8.0	140
1/30/2009	14	Formaldehyde	60	30.10	2.2	60
1/30/2009	15	Acetic Acid	60	24.00	10	170
1/30/2009	15	Formaldehyde	60	30.20	3.7	100
1/30/2009	16	Acetic Acid	60	24.10	ND	ND
1/30/2009	16	Formaldehyde	60	29.90	ND	ND
1/30/2009	17	Acetic Acid	NA	NA	ND	ND
1/30/2009	17	Formaldehyde	NA	NA	ND	ND
2/2/2009	1	Acetic Acid	60	24.40	17	280
2/2/2009	1	Formaldehyde	60	29.60	8.9	250
2/2/2009	2	Acetic Acid	60	25.00	15	240
2/2/2009	2	Formaldehyde	60	29.50	3.4	94
2/2/2009	3	Acetic Acid	60	24.30	7.0	120
2/2/2009	3	Formaldehyde	60	29.40	4.3	120
2/2/2009	4	Acetic Acid	60	24.50	8.0	130
2/2/2009	4	Formaldehyde	60	29.20	4.1	110
2/2/2009	5	Acetic Acid	60	24.80	8.0	130
2/2/2009	5	Formaldehyde	60	29.50	3.8	110
2/2/2009	6	Acetaldehyde	60	29.50	0.20	3.8
2/2/2009	6	Acetic Acid	60	23.90	8.0	140
2/2/2009	6	Formaldehyde	60	29.50	5.5	150
2/2/2009	7	Acetic Acid	60	24.10	12	200

Date	Trailer	Analyte	Sample Duration (minutes)	Sample Volume (liters)	Sample Mass (µg)	Concentration (ppb)
2/2/2009	7	Formaldehyde	60	29.60	5.0	140
2/2/2009	8	Acetic Acid	60	24.40	9.0	150
2/2/2009	8	Formaldehyde	60	29.30	2.0	56
2/2/2009	9	Acetic Acid	60	24.40	ND	ND
2/2/2009	9	Formaldehyde	60	29.40	1.3	36
2/2/2009	10	Acetaldehyde	60	29.30	0.3	5.7
2/2/2009	10	Acetic Acid	60	24.40	4.0	67
2/2/2009	10	Formaldehyde	60	29.30	3.4	94
2/2/2009	11	Acetaldehyde	60	29.80	0.30	5.6
2/2/2009	11	Acetic Acid	60	24.30	13	220
2/2/2009	11	Formaldehyde	60	29.80	9.7	270
2/2/2009	12	Acetaldehyde	60	29.80	0.20	3.7
2/2/2009	12	Acetic Acid	60	24.50	5.0	83
2/2/2009	12	Formaldehyde	60	29.80	2.4	66
2/2/2009	13	Acetaldehyde	60	29.70	0.40	7.5
2/2/2009	13	Acetic Acid	60	24.70	4.0	66
2/2/2009	13	Formaldehyde	60	29.70	2.5	68
2/2/2009	14	Acetic Acid	60	24.40	3.0	50
2/2/2009	14	Formaldehyde	60	29.70	2.7	74
2/2/2009	15	Acetaldehyde	60	30.20	0.20	3.7
2/2/2009	15	Formaldehyde	60	30.20	3.8	100
2/2/2009	16	Acetic Acid	60	24.00	ND	ND
2/2/2009	16	Formaldehyde	60	29.60	ND	ND
2/2/2009	17	Acetic Acid	NA	NA	ND	ND
2/2/2009	17	Formaldehyde	NA	NA	ND	ND
2/4/2009	1	Formaldehyde	60	29.70	6.8	190
2/4/2009	2	Formaldehyde	60	28.80	2.6	73
2/4/2009	3	Formaldehyde	60	29.20	2.7	75
2/4/2009	4	Formaldehyde	60	29.70	2.8	77
2/4/2009	5	Formaldehyde	60	29.80	3.3	90
2/4/2009	6	Formaldehyde	60	29.90	3.5	95
2/4/2009	7	Formaldehyde	60	29.70	2.7	74
2/4/2009	8	Formaldehyde	60	29.60	2.3	63
2/4/2009	9	Formaldehyde	60	29.80	0.50	14
2/4/2009	10	Formaldehyde	60	29.90	2.5	68
2/4/2009	11	Acetaldehyde	60	30.10	0.30	5.5
2/4/2009	11	Formaldehyde	60	30.10	7.7	210
2/4/2009	12	Formaldehyde	60	30.20	1.5	41
2/4/2009	13	Acetaldehyde	60	30.30	0.20	3.7
2/4/2009	13	Formaldehyde	60	30.30	1.6	43
2/4/2009	14	Formaldehyde	60	29.90	1.7	46
2/4/2009	15	Formaldehyde	60	29.80	2.5	68
2/4/2009	16	Formaldehyde	60	30.00	ND	ND
2/4/2009	17	Formaldehyde	NA	NA	ND	ND

Date	Trailer	Analyte	Sample Duration (minutes)	Sample Volume (liters)	Sample Mass (μg)	Concentration (ppb)
2/4/2009	18	Formaldehyde	0	NA	ND	ND
2/6/2009	1	Formaldehyde	60	30.90	13	340
2/6/2009	2	Acetaldehyde	61	30.90	0.30	5.4
2/6/2009	2	Formaldehyde	61	30.90	5.8	150
2/6/2009	3	Formaldehyde	60	30.80	6.5	170
2/6/2009	4	Acetaldehyde	0	31.10	0.20	3.6
2/6/2009	4	Formaldehyde	0	31.10	6.9	180
2/6/2009	5	Acetaldehyde	60	30.80	0.20	3.6
2/6/2009	5	Formaldehyde	60	30.80	8.1	210
2/6/2009	6	Acetaldehyde	60	30.50	0.30	5.5
2/6/2009	6	Formaldehyde	60	30.50	9.0	240
2/6/2009	7	Acetaldehyde	60	30.50	0.20	3.6
2/6/2009	7	Formaldehyde	60	30.50	6.8	180
2/6/2009	8	Acetaldehyde	61	30.80	0.20	3.6
2/6/2009	8	Formaldehyde	61	30.80	4.8	130
2/6/2009	9	Formaldehyde	61	33.00	1.5	37
2/6/2009	10	Acetaldehyde	60	32.20	0.50	8.6
2/6/2009	10	Formaldehyde	60	32.20	6.8	170
2/6/2009	11	Acetaldehyde	60	31.50	0.50	8.8
2/6/2009	11	Formaldehyde	60	31.50	17	440
2/6/2009	12	Acetaldehyde	60	30.60	0.30	5.4
2/6/2009	12	Formaldehyde	60	30.60	3.8	100
2/6/2009	13	Acetaldehyde	60	30.80	0.40	7.2
2/6/2009	13	Formaldehyde	60	30.80	3.9	100
2/6/2009	14	Acetaldehyde	60	31.10	0.20	3.6
2/6/2009	14	Formaldehyde	60	31.10	4.5	120
2/6/2009	15	Acetaldehyde	60	31.50	0.20	3.5
2/6/2009	15	Formaldehyde	60	31.50	6.0	160
2/6/2009	16	Formaldehyde	60	31.40	ND	ND
2/6/2009	17	Formaldehyde	NA	NA	ND	ND
2/9/2009	1	Acetic Acid	65	26.70	13	200
2/9/2009	1	Formaldehyde	0	31.50	9.8	250
2/9/2009	2	Acetic Acid	65	26.40	11	170
2/9/2009	2	Formaldehyde	0	13.50	2.2	130
2/9/2009	3	Acetic Acid	69	28.30	12	170
2/9/2009	3	Formaldehyde	0	13.30	2.2	130
2/9/2009	4	Acetic Acid	65	26.50	11	170
2/9/2009	4	Formaldehyde	0	12.70	2.5	160
2/9/2009	5	Acetaldehyde	49	24.90	0.20	4.5
2/9/2009	5	Acetic Acid	66	27.00	12	180
2/9/2009	5	Formaldehyde	49	24.90	6.2	200
2/9/2009	6	Acetic Acid	69	28.30	8.5	120
2/9/2009	6	Formaldehyde	45	23.50	3.7	130
2/9/2009	7	Acetic Acid	67	27.50	9.4	140

Date	Trailer	Analyte	Sample Duration (minutes)	Sample Volume (liters)	Sample Mass (μg)	Concentration (ppb)
2/9/2009	7	Formaldehyde	67	33.90	6.9	170
2/9/2009	8	Acetaldehyde	68	34.90	0.40	6.4
2/9/2009	8	Acetic Acid	68	27.60	7.9	120
2/9/2009	8	Formaldehyde	68	34.90	4.1	96
2/9/2009	9	Acetic Acid	69	28.00	3.7	53
2/9/2009	9	Formaldehyde	0	30.20	1.6	430
2/9/2009	10	Acetaldehyde	65	32.90	0.6	10
2/9/2009	10	Acetic Acid	65	26.30	5.8	90
2/9/2009	10	Formaldehyde	65	32.90	6.3	160
2/9/2009	11	Acetaldehyde	64	32.90	0.40	6.7
2/9/2009	11	Acetic Acid	64	25.90	16	250
2/9/2009	11	Formaldehyde	64	32.90	14	350
2/9/2009	12	Acetaldehyde	67	34.20	0.30	4.9
2/9/2009	12	Acetic Acid	67	26.80	4.7	71
2/9/2009	12	Formaldehyde	67	34.20	3.2	76
2/9/2009	13	Acetaldehyde	65	33.10	0.50	8.4
2/9/2009	13	Acetic Acid	65	26.20	7.1	110
2/9/2009	13	Formaldehyde	65	33.10	3.7	91
2/9/2009	14	Acetic Acid	67	26.90	7.5	110
2/9/2009	14	Formaldehyde	67	34.10	3.5	84
2/9/2009	15	Acetaldehyde	68	34.70	0.20	3.2
2/9/2009	15	Acetic Acid	68	27.30	8.9	130
2/9/2009	15	Formaldehyde	68	34.70	6.6	160
2/9/2009	16	Acetic Acid	69	27.80	ND	ND
2/9/2009	16	Formaldehyde	69	35.20	ND	ND
2/9/2009	17	Acetic Acid	NA	NA	ND	ND
2/9/2009	17	Formaldehyde	NA	NA	ND	ND
2/12/2009	1	Acetaldehyde	56	28.90	0.30	5.8
2/12/2009	1	Formaldehyde	56	28.90	16	450
2/12/2009	2	Acetaldehyde	40	20.80	0.20	5.3
2/12/2009	2	Formaldehyde	40	20.80	4.7	180
2/12/2009	3	Formaldehyde	41	20.90	5.1	200
2/12/2009	4	Acetaldehyde	41	21.20	0.20	5.2
2/12/2009	4	Formaldehyde	41	21.20	5.4	210
2/12/2009	5	Acetaldehyde	60	30.50	0.30	5.5
2/12/2009	5	Formaldehyde	60	30.50	9.0	240
2/12/2009	6	Acetaldehyde	60	30.60	0.30	5.4
2/12/2009	6	Formaldehyde	60	30.60	11	290
2/12/2009	7	Acetaldehyde	60	31.50	0.30	5.3
2/12/2009	7	Formaldehyde	60	31.50	8.4	220
2/12/2009	8	Acetaldehyde	60	31.20	0.30	5.3
2/12/2009	8	Formaldehyde	60	31.20	5.7	150
2/12/2009	9	Acetaldehyde	60	29.90	0.20	3.7
2/12/2009	9	Formaldehyde	60	29.90	1.7	46

Date	Trailer	Analyte	Sample Duration (minutes)	Sample Volume (liters)	Sample Mass (μg)	Concentration (ppb)
2/12/2009	10	Acetaldehyde	61	31.10	0.70	13
2/12/2009	10	Formaldehyde	61	31.10	8.1	210
2/12/2009	11	Acetaldehyde	60	30.30	0.40	7.3
2/12/2009	11	Formaldehyde	60	30.30	18	480
2/12/2009	12	Acetaldehyde	60	30.80	0.40	7.2
2/12/2009	12	Formaldehyde	60	30.80	4.0	110
2/12/2009	13	Acetaldehyde	60	30.70	0.60	11
2/12/2009	13	Formaldehyde	60	30.70	4.8	130
2/12/2009	14	Acetaldehyde	60	30.70	0.20	3.6
2/12/2009	14	Formaldehyde	60	30.70	4.9	130
2/12/2009	15	Acetaldehyde	60	30.80	0.20	3.6
2/12/2009	15	Formaldehyde	60	30.80	6.9	180
2/12/2009	16	Formaldehyde	0	32.00	ND	ND
2/12/2009	17	Formaldehyde	NA	NA	ND	ND
2/17/2009	1	Acetic Acid	60	24.20	8.0	140
2/17/2009	1	Formaldehyde	60	31.00	14	370
2/17/2009	2	Acetic Acid	61	24.30	6.0	100
2/17/2009	2	Formaldehyde	61	30.80	4.6	120
2/17/2009	3	Acetic Acid	60	23.70	4.0	69
2/17/2009	3	Formaldehyde	60	30.60	6.0	160
2/17/2009	4	Acetic Acid	60	23.80	8.0	140
2/17/2009	4	Formaldehyde	60	30.70	5.3	140
2/17/2009	5	Acetic Acid	60	24.00	7.0	120
2/17/2009	5	Formaldehyde	60	30.70	6.6	180
2/17/2009	6	Acetaldehyde	60	30.40	0.20	3.7
2/17/2009	6	Acetic Acid	60	23.50	4.0	69
2/17/2009	6	Formaldehyde	60	30.40	7.7	210
2/17/2009	7	Acetic Acid	60	24.00	4.0	68
2/17/2009	7	Formaldehyde	60	30.60	5.8	150
2/17/2009	8	Acetaldehyde	60	31.30	0.20	3.5
2/17/2009	8	Acetic Acid	60	23.70	5.0	86
2/17/2009	8	Formaldehyde	60	31.30	5.0	130
2/17/2009	9	Acetic Acid	60	23.60	2.0	34
2/17/2009	9	Formaldehyde	60	30.50	1.4	37
2/17/2009	10	Acetaldehyde	61	31.00	0.50	9.0
2/17/2009	10	Acetic Acid	61	23.80	5.0	86
2/17/2009	10	Formaldehyde	61	31.00	6.2	160
2/17/2009	11	Acetaldehyde	60	31.00	0.40	7.2
2/17/2009	11	Acetic Acid	60	23.90	8.0	140
2/17/2009	11	Formaldehyde	60	31.00	16	420
2/17/2009	12	Acetaldehyde	60	30.70	0.20	3.6
2/17/2009	12	Acetic Acid	60	23.90	ND	ND
2/17/2009	12	Formaldehyde	60	30.70	3.7	98
2/17/2009	13	Acetaldehyde	60	30.60	0.40	7.2

Date	Trailer	Analyte	Sample Duration (minutes)	Sample Volume (liters)	Sample Mass (μg)	Concentration (ppb)
2/17/2009	13	Acetic Acid	60	23.70	ND	ND
2/17/2009	13	Formaldehyde	60	30.60	3.8	100
2/17/2009	14	Acetaldehyde	61	31.50	0.30	5.3
2/17/2009	14	Acetic Acid	61	24.90	3.0	49
2/17/2009	14	Formaldehyde	61	31.50	3.9	100
2/17/2009	15	Acetaldehyde	60	31.00	0.20	3.6
2/17/2009	15	Acetic Acid	60	24.00	4.0	68
2/17/2009	15	Formaldehyde	60	31.00	5.4	140
2/17/2009	16	Acetic Acid	60	23.90	ND	ND
2/17/2009	16	Formaldehyde	60	31.00	ND	ND
2/17/2009	17	Acetic Acid	NA	NA	ND	ND
2/17/2009	17	Formaldehyde	NA	NA	ND	ND
2/17/2009	18	Formaldehyde	0	NA	ND	ND
2/20/2009	1	Formaldehyde	60	30.00	8.9	240
2/20/2009	2	Formaldehyde	60	29.60	3.5	96
2/20/2009	3	Formaldehyde	60	29.80	3.7	100
2/20/2009	4	Formaldehyde	60	30.00	3.8	100
2/20/2009	5	Formaldehyde	60	29.80	4.8	130
2/20/2009	6	Formaldehyde	60	29.70	5.1	140
2/20/2009	7	Formaldehyde	60	29.90	4.6	130
2/20/2009	8	Formaldehyde	61	30.90	4.1	110
2/20/2009	9	Formaldehyde	61	30.30	1.0	27
2/20/2009	10	Acetaldehyde	60	30.00	0.30	5.6
2/20/2009	10	Formaldehyde	60	30.00	4.2	110
2/20/2009	11	Acetaldehyde	61	30.50	0.70	13
2/20/2009	11	Formaldehyde	61	30.50	12	320
2/20/2009	12	Formaldehyde	61	30.70	2.5	66
2/20/2009	13	Acetaldehyde	61	30.50	0.3	5.5
2/20/2009	13	Formaldehyde	61	30.50	2.7	72
2/20/2009	14	Formaldehyde	60	30.20	2.9	78
2/20/2009	15	Formaldehyde	60	30.40	4.0	110
2/20/2009	16	Formaldehyde	61	31.30	ND	ND
2/20/2009	17	Formaldehyde	NA	NA	ND	ND
2/23/2009	1	Acetic Acid	60	23.60	7.0	120
2/23/2009	1	Formaldehyde	60	30.70	9.2	240
2/23/2009	2	Acetic Acid	60	23.80	8.0	140
2/23/2009	2	Formaldehyde	60	30.90	3.4	90
2/23/2009	3	Acetic Acid	60	24.00	5.0	85
2/23/2009	3	Formaldehyde	60	30.40	3.9	110
2/23/2009	4	Acetic Acid	60	23.80	7.0	120
2/23/2009	4	Formaldehyde	60	30.50	3.7	99
2/23/2009	5	Acetic Acid	60	24.30	7.0	120
2/23/2009	5	Formaldehyde	60	31.40	4.4	110
2/23/2009	6	Acetic Acid	60	24.60	6.0	99

Date	Trailer	Analyte	Sample Duration (minutes)	Sample Volume (liters)	Sample Mass (μg)	Concentration (ppb)
2/23/2009	6	Formaldehyde	60	30.50	5.4	140
2/23/2009	7	Acetic Acid	60	23.50	6.0	100
2/23/2009	7	Formaldehyde	60	30.60	4.2	110
2/23/2009	8	Acetaldehyde	60	30.20	0.40	7.3
2/23/2009	8	Acetic Acid	60	24.30	9.0	150
2/23/2009	8	Formaldehyde	60	30.20	3.6	97
2/23/2009	9	Acetic Acid	60	24.20	2.0	34
2/23/2009	9	Formaldehyde	60	30.50	0.90	24
2/23/2009	10	Acetaldehyde	60	30.60	0.20	3.6
2/23/2009	10	Acetic Acid	60	24.20	5.0	84
2/23/2009	10	Formaldehyde	60	30.60	3.6	96
2/23/2009	11	Acetaldehyde	60	30.40	0.70	13
2/23/2009	11	Acetic Acid	60	24.40	13	220
2/23/2009	11	Formaldehyde	60	30.40	11	290
2/23/2009	12	Acetic Acid	60	24.10	3.0	51
2/23/2009	12	Formaldehyde	60	30.60	2.3	61
2/23/2009	13	Acetaldehyde	60	30.40	0.20	3.7
2/23/2009	13	Acetic Acid	60	24.20	4.0	67
2/23/2009	13	Formaldehyde	60	30.40	2.2	59
2/23/2009	14	Acetic Acid	60	24.20	6.0	100
2/23/2009	14	Formaldehyde	60	30.30	2.4	65
2/23/2009	15	Acetic Acid	60	24.20	6.0	100
2/23/2009	15	Formaldehyde	60	30.50	3.3	88
2/23/2009	16	Acetic Acid	60	24.50	ND	ND
2/23/2009	16	Formaldehyde	60	30.10	ND	ND
2/23/2009	17	Acetic Acid	NA	NA	ND	ND
2/23/2009	17	Formaldehyde	NA	NA	ND	ND
2/26/2009	1	Formaldehyde	24	12.00	6.5	440
2/26/2009	2	Formaldehyde	60	29.70	5.7	160
2/26/2009	3	Formaldehyde	42	21.30	4.8	180
2/26/2009	4	Formaldehyde	52	26.30	6.6	200
2/26/2009	5	Formaldehyde	61	31.30	8.4	220
2/26/2009	6	Formaldehyde	48	24.40	7.2	240
2/26/2009	7	Acetaldehyde	60	30.50	0.20	3.6
2/26/2009	7	Formaldehyde	60	30.50	8.2	220
2/26/2009	8	Formaldehyde	62	31.30	5.4	140
2/26/2009	9	Formaldehyde	39	22.10	1.9	70
2/26/2009	10	Acetaldehyde	60	30.90	0.70	13
2/26/2009	10	Formaldehyde	60	30.90	7.4	200
2/26/2009	11	Acetaldehyde	62	31.90	0.60	11
2/26/2009	11	Formaldehyde	62	31.90	22	502
2/26/2009	12	Acetaldehyde	60	31.20	0.30	5.3
2/26/2009	12	Formaldehyde	60	31.20	4.3	110
2/26/2009	13	Acetaldehyde	60	30.90	0.50	9.0

Date	Trailer	Analyte	Sample Duration (minutes)	Sample Volume (liters)	Sample Mass (µg)	Concentration (ppb)
2/26/2009	13	Formaldehyde	60	30.90	4.4	120
2/26/2009	14	Acetaldehyde	60	30.60	0.20	3.6
2/26/2009	14	Formaldehyde	60	30.60	5.0	130
2/26/2009	15	Formaldehyde	60	30.70	6.1	160
2/26/2009	16	Formaldehyde	60	31.20	ND	ND
2/26/2009	17	Formaldehyde	0	NA	ND	ND
3/2/2009	1	Acetic Acid	60	23.00	6.0	110
3/2/2009	1	Formaldehyde	60	29.30	5.1	140
3/2/2009	2	Acetic Acid	60	23.30	6.0	110
3/2/2009	2	Formaldehyde	60	29.50	2.2	61
3/2/2009	4	Acetic Acid	60	23.60	5.0	86
3/2/2009	4	Formaldehyde	47	22.50	1.8	65
3/2/2009	5	Acetic Acid	60	23.80	6.0	100
3/2/2009	5	Formaldehyde	60	29.70	3.7	100
3/2/2009	6	Acetic Acid	60	23.80	5.0	86
3/2/2009	6	Formaldehyde	60	29.70	3.7	100
3/2/2009	7	Acetic Acid	60	23.80	6.0	100
3/2/2009	7	Formaldehyde	60	30.00	3.0	82
3/2/2009	8	Acetic Acid	60	23.90	8.0	140
3/2/2009	8	Formaldehyde	60	29.90	3.1	85
3/2/2009	9	Acetic Acid	60	24.30	ND	ND
3/2/2009	9	Formaldehyde	60	29.60	0.50	14
3/2/2009	10	Acetic Acid	60	23.80	2.0	34
3/2/2009	10	Formaldehyde	60	29.60	2.0	55
3/2/2009	11	Acetaldehyde	60	29.70	0.40	7.5
3/2/2009	11	Acetic Acid	60	24.00	9.0	150
3/2/2009	11	Formaldehyde	60	29.70	7.1	200
3/2/2009	12	Acetic Acid	60	23.90	2.0	34
3/2/2009	12	Formaldehyde	60	29.80	1.6	44
3/2/2009	13	Acetaldehyde	60	29.90	0.20	3.7
3/2/2009	13	Acetic Acid	60	23.50	2.0	35
3/2/2009	13	Formaldehyde	60	29.90	1.9	52
3/2/2009	14	Acetic Acid	60	23.90	3.0	51
3/2/2009	14	Formaldehyde	60	29.70	2.0	55
3/2/2009	15	Acetic Acid	60	24.10	5.0	85
3/2/2009	15	Formaldehyde	60	29.90	2.3	63
3/2/2009	16	Acetic Acid	60	24.10	ND	ND
3/2/2009	16	Formaldehyde	60	30.20	ND	ND
3/2/2009	17	Acetic Acid	NA	NA	ND	ND
3/2/2009	17	Formaldehyde	NA	NA	ND	ND
3/2/2009	18	Acetic Acid	0	NA	ND	ND
3/5/2009	1	Formaldehyde	60	30.30	13	350
3/5/2009	2	Formaldehyde	60	30.10	5.9	160
3/5/2009	4	Formaldehyde	60	30.30	6.5	180

Date	Trailer	Analyte	Sample Duration (minutes)	Sample Volume (liters)	Sample Mass (µg)	Concentration (ppb)
3/5/2009	5	Formaldehyde	60	30.10	7.1	190
3/5/2009	6	Acetaldehyde	60	30.60	0.30	5.4
3/5/2009	6	Formaldehyde	60	30.60	9.5	250
3/5/2009	7	Formaldehyde	60	30.30	5.7	150
3/5/2009	8	Acetaldehyde	60	30.10	0.20	3.7
3/5/2009	8	Formaldehyde	60	30.10	5.9	160
3/5/2009	9	Formaldehyde	60	30.30	1.8	48
3/5/2009	10	Acetaldehyde	60	30.10	0.50	9.2
3/5/2009	10	Formaldehyde	60	30.10	6.0	160
3/5/2009	11	Acetaldehyde	60	30.30	0.50	9.2
3/5/2009	11	Formaldehyde	60	30.30	19	510
3/5/2009	12	Acetaldehyde	60	30.20	0.20	3.7
3/5/2009	12	Formaldehyde	60	30.20	3.2	86
3/5/2009	13	Acetaldehyde	60	30.40	0.40	7.3
3/5/2009	13	Formaldehyde	60	30.40	3.4	91
3/5/2009	14	Acetaldehyde	60	30.30	0.20	3.7
3/5/2009	14	Formaldehyde	60	30.30	4.2	110
3/5/2009	15	Formaldehyde	60	30.40	5.3	140
3/5/2009	16	Formaldehyde	60	30.20	ND	ND
3/5/2009	17	Formaldehyde	NA	NA	ND	ND
3/9/2009	1	Acetaldehyde	60	30.90	0.30	5.4
3/9/2009	1	Acetic Acid	60	24.90	10	160
3/9/2009	1	Formaldehyde	60	30.90	19	500
3/9/2009	2	Acetaldehyde	60	30.60	0.20	3.6
3/9/2009	2	Acetic Acid	60	25.00	12	200
3/9/2009	2	Formaldehyde	60	30.60	7.1	190
3/9/2009	4	Acetaldehyde	60	30.50	0.50	9.1
3/9/2009	4	Acetic Acid	60	25.10	11	180
3/9/2009	4	Formaldehyde	60	30.50	8.3	220
3/9/2009	5	Acetaldehyde	60	31.30	0.20	3.5
3/9/2009	5	Acetic Acid	60	25.00	11	180
3/9/2009	5	Formaldehyde	60	31.30	9.4	250
3/9/2009	6	Acetaldehyde	60	31.30	0.30	5.3
3/9/2009	6	Acetic Acid	60	25.10	10	160
3/9/2009	6	Formaldehyde	60	31.30	12	310
3/9/2009	7	Acetaldehyde	60	31.80	0.30	5.2
3/9/2009	7	Acetic Acid	60	25.00	5.0	81
3/9/2009	7	Formaldehyde	60	31.80	9.0	230
3/9/2009	8	Acetaldehyde	60	31.80	0.20	3.5
3/9/2009	8	Acetic Acid	60	25.20	8.0	130
3/9/2009	8	Formaldehyde	60	31.80	7.6	200
3/9/2009	9	Acetic Acid	60	24.80	3.0	49
3/9/2009	9	Formaldehyde	60	31.30	3.2	83
3/9/2009	10	Acetaldehyde	60	31.40	0.90	16

Date	Trailer	Analyte	Sample Duration (minutes)	Sample Volume (liters)	Sample Mass (µg)	Concentration (ppb)
3/9/2009	10	Acetic Acid	60	25.00	3.0	49
3/9/2009	10	Formaldehyde	60	31.40	9.1	240
3/9/2009	11	Acetaldehyde	60	31.60	0.70	12
3/9/2009	11	Acetic Acid	60	24.70	9.0	150
3/9/2009	11	Formaldehyde	60	31.60	18	460
3/9/2009	12	Acetaldehyde	60	31.10	0.40	7.1
3/9/2009	12	Acetic Acid	60	24.90	5.0	82
3/9/2009	12	Formaldehyde	60	31.10	5.2	140
3/9/2009	13	Acetaldehyde	60	31.10	0.70	13
3/9/2009	13	Acetic Acid	60	25.10	6.0	97
3/9/2009	13	Formaldehyde	60	31.10	5.3	140
3/9/2009	14	Acetaldehyde	60	31.10	0.20	3.6
3/9/2009	14	Acetic Acid	60	24.70	ND	ND
3/9/2009	14	Formaldehyde	60	31.10	6.5	170
3/9/2009	15	Acetic Acid	61	25.40	ND	ND
3/9/2009	15	Formaldehyde	61	31.50	6.8	180
3/9/2009	16	Acetic Acid	60	24.90	ND	ND
3/9/2009	16	Formaldehyde	60	31.40	ND	ND
3/9/2009	17	Acetic Acid	NA	NA	ND	ND
3/9/2009	17	Formaldehyde	NA	NA	ND	ND
3/12/2009	1	Acetaldehyde	60	30.40	0.20	3.7
3/12/2009	1	Formaldehyde	60	30.40	19	510
3/12/2009	2	Acetaldehyde	60	29.90	0.20	3.7
3/12/2009	2	Formaldehyde	60	29.90	8.0	220
3/12/2009	4	Formaldehyde	60	30.70	8.2	220
3/12/2009	5	Formaldehyde	60	30.60	10	270
3/12/2009	6	Acetaldehyde	60	30.60	0.30	5.4
3/12/2009	6	Formaldehyde	60	30.60	12	320
3/12/2009	7	Formaldehyde	60	30.10	9.2	250
3/12/2009	8	Formaldehyde	60	30.40	9.4	250
3/12/2009	9	Formaldehyde	60	30.10	2.1	57
3/12/2009	10	Acetaldehyde	60	30.60	0.60	11
3/12/2009	10	Formaldehyde	60	30.60	8.9	240
3/12/2009	11	Acetaldehyde	60	30.50	0.60	11
3/12/2009	11	Formaldehyde	60	30.50	19	510
3/12/2009	12	Acetaldehyde	60	29.90	0.30	5.6
3/12/2009	12	Formaldehyde	60	29.90	4.5	120
3/12/2009	13	Acetaldehyde	60	30.60	0.60	11
3/12/2009	13	Formaldehyde	60	30.60	5.0	130
3/12/2009	14	Acetaldehyde	60	30.60	0.20	3.6
3/12/2009	14	Formaldehyde	60	30.60	6.0	160
3/12/2009	15	Acetaldehyde	60	30.70	0.20	3.6
3/12/2009	15	Formaldehyde	60	30.70	7.3	190
3/12/2009	16	Formaldehyde	60	31.30	ND	ND

Date	Trailer	Analyte	Sample Duration (minutes)	Sample Volume (liters)	Sample Mass (µg)	Concentration (ppb)
3/12/2009	17	Formaldehyde	NA	NA	ND	ND
3/17/2009	1	Acetaldehyde	60	30.00	0.20	3.7
3/17/2009	1	Acetic Acid	60	23.90	16	270
3/17/2009	1	Formaldehyde	60	30.00	20	540
3/17/2009	2	Acetaldehyde	60	30.30	0.20	3.7
3/17/2009	2	Acetic Acid	60	23.80	14	240
3/17/2009	2	Formaldehyde	60	30.30	7.5	200
3/17/2009	4	Acetaldehyde	60	30.50	0.30	5.5
3/17/2009	4	Acetic Acid	60	24.30	15	250
3/17/2009	4	Formaldehyde	60	30.50	8.9	240
3/17/2009	5	Acetaldehyde	60	30.40	0.20	3.6
3/17/2009	5	Acetic Acid	60	24.00	14	240
3/17/2009	5	Formaldehyde	60	30.40	11	290
3/17/2009	6	Acetaldehyde	60	30.60	0.30	5.4
3/17/2009	6	Acetic Acid	60	24.30	8.0	130
3/17/2009	6	Formaldehyde	60	30.60	13	350
3/17/2009	7	Acetaldehyde	60	30.20	0.30	5.5
3/17/2009	7	Acetic Acid	60	24.30	3.0	50
3/17/2009	7	Formaldehyde	60	30.20	7.9	220
3/17/2009	8	Acetaldehyde	60	29.90	0.30	5.6
3/17/2009	8	Acetic Acid	60	24.90	8.0	130
3/17/2009	8	Formaldehyde	60	29.90	8.3	230
3/17/2009	9	Acetic Acid	60	24.40	3.0	50
3/17/2009	9	Formaldehyde	60	30.60	3.1	82
3/17/2009	10	Acetaldehyde	60	30.70	1.0	18
3/17/2009	10	Acetic Acid	60	24.30	5.0	84
3/17/2009	10	Formaldehyde	60	30.70	10	270
3/17/2009	11	Acetaldehyde	60	30.50	0.50	9.1
3/17/2009	11	Acetic Acid	60	24.40	10	170
3/17/2009	11	Formaldehyde	60	30.50	21	560
3/17/2009	12	Acetaldehyde	60	31.00	0.40	7.2
3/17/2009	12	Acetic Acid	60	24.40	4.0	67
3/17/2009	12	Formaldehyde	60	31.00	5.1	130
3/17/2009	13	Acetaldehyde	60	31.10	0.70	13
3/17/2009	13	Acetic Acid	60	24.50	4.0	67
3/17/2009	13	Formaldehyde	60	31.10	5.8	150
3/17/2009	14	Acetaldehyde	60	30.80	0.30	5.4
3/17/2009	14	Acetic Acid	60	24.40	8.0	130
3/17/2009	14	Formaldehyde	60	30.80	6.5	170
3/17/2009	15	Acetaldehyde	60	30.60	0.20	3.6
3/17/2009	15	Acetic Acid	60	24.40	10	170
3/17/2009	15	Formaldehyde	60	30.60	7.1	190
3/17/2009	16	Acetic Acid	60	24.80	ND	ND
3/17/2009	16	Formaldehyde	60	31.60	ND	ND

Date	Trailer	Analyte	Sample Duration (minutes)	Sample Volume (liters)	Sample Mass (μg)	Concentration (ppb)
3/17/2009	17	Acetic Acid	NA	NA	ND	ND
3/17/2009	17	Formaldehyde	NA	NA	ND	ND
3/19/2009	1	Acetaldehyde	60	29.80	0.20	3.7
3/19/2009	1	Formaldehyde	60	29.80	20	550
3/19/2009	2	Acetaldehyde	60	31.70	0.30	5.3
3/19/2009	2	Formaldehyde	60	31.70	8	210
3/19/2009	4	Acetaldehyde	60	31.10	0.30	5.4
3/19/2009	4	Formaldehyde	60	31.10	9.6	250
3/19/2009	5	Acetaldehyde	60	31.00	0.20	3.6
3/19/2009	5	Formaldehyde	60	31.00	11	290
3/19/2009	6	Acetaldehyde	60	31.60	0.30	5.3
3/19/2009	6	Formaldehyde	60	31.60	13	340
3/19/2009	7	Acetaldehyde	60	30.90	0.30	5.4
3/19/2009	7	Formaldehyde	60	30.90	8.5	220
3/19/2009	8	Acetaldehyde	60	31.00	0.30	5.4
3/19/2009	8	Formaldehyde	60	31.00	10	260
3/19/2009	9	Formaldehyde	60	30.50	2.8	75
3/19/2009	10	Acetaldehyde	60	31.50	1.0	18
3/19/2009	10	Formaldehyde	60	31.50	10	260
3/19/2009	11	Acetaldehyde	60	31.40	0.70	12
3/19/2009	11	Formaldehyde	60	31.40	21	550
3/19/2009	12	Acetaldehyde	60	31.40	0.50	8.8
3/19/2009	12	Formaldehyde	60	31.40	5.3	140
3/19/2009	13	Acetaldehyde	60	30.90	0.70	13
3/19/2009	13	Formaldehyde	60	30.90	5.5	150
3/19/2009	14	Acetaldehyde	60	31.10	0.30	5.4
3/19/2009	14	Formaldehyde	60	31.10	7.6	200
3/19/2009	15	Acetaldehyde	60	31.30	0.30	5.3
3/19/2009	15	Formaldehyde	60	31.30	7.3	190
3/19/2009	16	Formaldehyde	60	31.20	ND	ND
3/19/2009	17	Formaldehyde	NA	NA	ND	ND
3/23/2009	1	Acetaldehyde	60	30.50	0.20	3.6
3/23/2009	1	Acetic Acid	60	23.80	12	210
3/23/2009	1	Formaldehyde	60	30.50	20	530
3/23/2009	2	Acetaldehyde	60	30.20	0.30	5.5
3/23/2009	2	Acetic Acid	60	24.00	12	200
3/23/2009	2	Formaldehyde	60	30.20	7.7	210
3/23/2009	4	Acetaldehyde	60	30.30	0.30	5.5
3/23/2009	4	Acetic Acid	60	24.00	12	200
3/23/2009	4	Formaldehyde	60	30.30	8.4	230
3/23/2009	5	Acetaldehyde	60	30.90	0.30	5.4
3/23/2009	5	Acetic Acid	60	24.10	9.0	150
3/23/2009	5	Formaldehyde	60	30.90	9.9	260
3/23/2009	6	Acetaldehyde	60	30.80	0.40	7.2

Date	Trailer	Analyte	Sample Duration (minutes)	Sample Volume (liters)	Sample Mass (µg)	Concentration (ppb)
3/23/2009	6	Acetic Acid	60	24.20	8.0	140
3/23/2009	6	Formaldehyde	60	30.80	12	320
3/23/2009	7	Acetaldehyde	60	30.90	0.30	5.4
3/23/2009	7	Acetic Acid	60	24.30	6.0	100
3/23/2009	7	Formaldehyde	60	30.90	8.6	230
3/23/2009	8	Acetaldehyde	60	30.20	0.30	5.5
3/23/2009	8	Acetic Acid	60	25.00	9.0	150
3/23/2009	8	Formaldehyde	60	30.20	11	300
3/23/2009	9	Acetic Acid	60	24.40	ND	ND
3/23/2009	9	Formaldehyde	60	30.60	2.3	61
3/23/2009	10	Acetaldehyde	60	30.90	0.80	14
3/23/2009	10	Acetic Acid	60	24.10	4.0	68
3/23/2009	10	Formaldehyde	60	30.90	8.6	230
3/23/2009	11	Acetaldehyde	60	30.90	0.60	11
3/23/2009	11	Acetic Acid	60	24.30	14	240
3/23/2009	11	Formaldehyde	60	30.90	21	550
3/23/2009	12	Acetaldehyde	60	30.70	0.40	7.2
3/23/2009	12	Acetic Acid	60	24.40	8.0	130
3/23/2009	12	Formaldehyde	60	30.70	4.7	130
3/23/2009	13	Acetaldehyde	60	30.70	0.60	11
3/23/2009	13	Acetic Acid	60	24.70	4.0	66
3/23/2009	13	Formaldehyde	60	30.70	4.6	120
3/23/2009	14	Acetaldehyde	60	31.10	0.30	5.4
3/23/2009	14	Acetic Acid	60	24.60	7.0	120
3/23/2009	14	Formaldehyde	60	31.10	5.8	150
3/23/2009	15	Acetaldehyde	60	30.60	0.20	3.6
3/23/2009	15	Acetic Acid	60	24.50	7.0	120
3/23/2009	15	Formaldehyde	60	30.60	7.1	190
3/23/2009	16	Acetic Acid	60	24.40	ND	ND
3/23/2009	16	Formaldehyde	60	30.40	ND	ND
3/23/2009	17	Acetic Acid	NA	NA	ND	ND
3/23/2009	17	Formaldehyde	NA	NA	ND	ND
3/26/2009	1	Formaldehyde	60	30.40	18	480
3/26/2009	2	Formaldehyde	60	30.10	3.6	97
3/26/2009	4	Formaldehyde	60	29.80	3.9	110
3/26/2009	5	Formaldehyde	60	30.00	5.3	140
3/26/2009	6	Formaldehyde	60	30.00	3.2	87
3/26/2009	7	Formaldehyde	60	30.30	5.1	140
3/26/2009	8	Formaldehyde	60	29.90	5.1	140
3/26/2009	9	Formaldehyde	60	30.10	1.6	43
3/26/2009	10	Acetaldehyde	60	29.40	0.50	9.4
3/26/2009	10	Formaldehyde	60	29.40	5.0	140
3/26/2009	11	Acetaldehyde	60	30.10	0.30	5.5
3/26/2009	11	Formaldehyde	60	30.10	12	330

Date	Trailer	Analyte	Sample Duration (minutes)	Sample Volume (liters)	Sample Mass (μg)	Concentration (ppb)
3/26/2009	12	Acetaldehyde	60	30.00	0.30	5.5
3/26/2009	12	Formaldehyde	60	30.00	3.2	87
3/26/2009	13	Acetaldehyde	60	29.90	0.50	9.3
3/26/2009	13	Formaldehyde	60	29.90	4.0	110
3/26/2009	14	Formaldehyde	60	29.90	4.7	130
3/26/2009	15	Formaldehyde	60	30.40	5.7	150
3/26/2009	16	Formaldehyde	60	30.60	ND	ND
3/26/2009	17	Formaldehyde	NA	NA	ND	ND
3/30/2009	1	Formaldehyde	60	29.94	14	380
3/30/2009	1	Acetaldehyde	60	29.94	0.2	3.7
3/30/2009	1	Acetic Acid	60	23.90	13	220
3/30/2009	2	Formaldehyde	60	30.29	6.6	180
3/30/2009	2	Acetaldehyde	60	30.29	0.2	3.7
3/30/2009	2	Acetic Acid	60	23.94	13	220
3/30/2009	4	Formaldehyde	60	30.57	7.5	200
3/30/2009	4	Acetaldehyde	60	30.57	0.2	3.6
3/30/2009	4	Acetic Acid	60	24.01	11	190
3/30/2009	5	Formaldehyde	60	30.53	8.4	220
3/30/2009	5	Acetic Acid	60	24.02	14	240
3/30/2009	6	Formaldehyde	60	30.56	9.7	260
3/30/2009	6	Acetaldehyde	60	30.56	0.3	5.4
3/30/2009	6	Acetic Acid	60	24.53	8	130
3/30/2009	7	Formaldehyde	60	30.52	7.9	210
3/30/2009	7	Acetaldehyde	60	30.52	0.2	3.6
3/30/2009	7	Acetic Acid	60	24.65	13	220
3/30/2009	8	Formaldehyde	60	31.04	10	260
3/30/2009	8	Acetaldehyde	60	31.04	0.2	3.6
3/30/2009	8	Acetic Acid	60	24.21	12	200
3/30/2009	9	Formaldehyde	60	30.67	1.8	47
3/30/2009	9	Acetic Acid	60	24.21	ND	ND
3/30/2009	10	Formaldehyde	60	30.51	7.1	190
3/30/2009	10	Acetaldehyde	60	30.51	0.6	11
3/30/2009	10	Acetic Acid	60	24.56	7	120
3/30/2009	11	Formaldehyde	60	30.23	16	430
3/30/2009	11	Acetaldehyde	60	30.23	0.4	7.3
3/30/2009	11	Acetic Acid	60	24.17	18	300
3/30/2009	12	Formaldehyde	60	30.39	4.1	110
3/30/2009	12	Acetaldehyde	60	30.39	0.3	5.5
3/30/2009	12	Acetic Acid	60	24.32	5	84
3/30/2009	13	Formaldehyde	60	30.45	3.7	100
3/30/2009	13	Acetaldehyde	60	30.45	0.5	9.1
3/30/2009	13	Acetic Acid	60	24.46	5	83
3/30/2009	14	Formaldehyde	60	30.66	4.7	120
3/30/2009	14	Acetaldehyde	60	30.66	0.2	3.6

Date	Trailer	Analyte	Sample Duration (minutes)	Sample Volume (liters)	Sample Mass (µg)	Concentration (ppb)
3/30/2009	14	Acetic Acid	60	24.34	6	100
3/30/2009	15	Formaldehyde	60	30.65	5.1	140
3/30/2009	15	Acetic Acid	60	24.75	7	120
3/30/2009	16	Formaldehyde	60	30.75	ND	ND
3/30/2009	16	Acetic Acid	60	24.52	ND	ND
3/30/2009	17	Formaldehyde	NA	NA	ND	ND
3/30/2009	17	Acetic Acid	NA	NA	ND	ND
4/2/2009	1	Formaldehyde	105	51.68	25	390
4/2/2009	1	Acetaldehyde	105	51.68	0.3	3.2
4/2/2009	2	Formaldehyde	105	52.58	12	190
4/2/2009	2	Acetaldehyde	105	52.58	0.3	3.2
4/2/2009	4	Formaldehyde	105	51.93	15	240
4/2/2009	4	Acetaldehyde	105	51.93	0.3	3.2
4/2/2009	5	Formaldehyde	105	51.58	14	220
4/2/2009	5	Acetaldehyde	105	51.58	0.2	2.2
4/2/2009	6	Formaldehyde	105	52.20	19	300
4/2/2009	6	Acetaldehyde	105	52.20	0.3	3.2
4/2/2009	7	Formaldehyde	105	52.48	11	170
4/2/2009	7	Acetaldehyde	105	52.48	0.3	3.2
4/2/2009	8	Formaldehyde	105	51.44	18	280
4/2/2009	8	Acetaldehyde	105	51.44	0.3	3.2
4/2/2009	9	Formaldehyde	105	49.88	4.2	69
4/2/2009	10	Formaldehyde	107	52.88	15	230
4/2/2009	10	Acetaldehyde	107	52.88	1.2	13
4/2/2009	11	Formaldehyde	105	52.26	29	450
4/2/2009	11	Acetaldehyde	105	52.26	0.6	6.4
4/2/2009	12	Formaldehyde	105	52.31	8.9	140
4/2/2009	12	Acetaldehyde	105	52.31	0.5	5.3
4/2/2009	13	Formaldehyde	105	46.04	7.9	140
4/2/2009	13	Acetaldehyde	105	46.04	0.8	9.6
4/2/2009	14	Formaldehyde	122	58.97	9.3	130
4/2/2009	14	Acetaldehyde	122	58.97	0.3	2.8
4/2/2009	15	Formaldehyde	105	52.55	10	150
4/2/2009	15	Acetaldehyde	105	52.55	0.2	2.1
4/2/2009	16	Formaldehyde	106	31.85	ND	ND
4/2/2009	17	Formaldehyde	NA	NA	ND	ND
4/6/2009	1	Formaldehyde	60	29.74	12	330
4/6/2009	1	Acetaldehyde	60	29.74	0.2	3.7
4/6/2009	1	Acetic Acid	60	24.04	8	140
4/6/2009	2	Formaldehyde	60	30.46	5.1	140
4/6/2009	2	Acetaldehyde	60	30.46	0.2	3.6
4/6/2009	2	Acetic Acid	60	23.83	9	150
4/6/2009	4	Formaldehyde	60	29.77	5.3	140
4/6/2009	4	Acetaldehyde	60	29.77	0.2	3.7

Date	Trailer	Analyte	Sample Duration (minutes)	Sample Volume (liters)	Sample Mass (µg)	Concentration (ppb)
4/6/2009	4	Acetic Acid	60	23.81	9	150
4/6/2009	5	Formaldehyde	60	29.64	5.8	160
4/6/2009	5	Acetic Acid	60	23.78	8	140
4/6/2009	6	Formaldehyde	60	30.49	8.1	220
4/6/2009	6	Acetaldehyde	60	30.49	0.3	5.5
4/6/2009	6	Acetic Acid	60	23.81	7	120
4/6/2009	7	Formaldehyde	60	29.74	7.7	210
4/6/2009	7	Acetaldehyde	60	29.74	0.2	3.7
4/6/2009	7	Acetic Acid	60	23.89	14	240
4/6/2009	8	Formaldehyde	60	29.72	9.4	260
4/6/2009	8	Acetaldehyde	60	29.72	0.2	3.7
4/6/2009	8	Acetic Acid	60	23.48	7	120
4/6/2009	9	Formaldehyde	60	30.18	1.1	30
4/6/2009	9	Acetic Acid	60	24.02	ND	ND
4/6/2009	10	Formaldehyde	60	29.94	5.7	160
4/6/2009	10	Acetaldehyde	60	29.94	0.5	9.3
4/6/2009	10	Acetic Acid	60	23.70	3	52
4/6/2009	11	Formaldehyde	60	29.86	14	380
4/6/2009	11	Acetaldehyde	60	29.86	0.5	9.3
4/6/2009	11	Acetic Acid	60	23.69	11	190
4/6/2009	12	Formaldehyde	60	30.08	3.3	89
4/6/2009	12	Acetaldehyde	60	30.08	0.3	5.5
4/6/2009	12	Acetic Acid	60	23.81	3	51
4/6/2009	13	Formaldehyde	60	30.50	3.3	88
4/6/2009	13	Acetaldehyde	60	30.50	0.4	7.3
4/6/2009	13	Acetic Acid	60	24.05	3	51
4/6/2009	14	Formaldehyde	60	30.36	4.5	120
4/6/2009	14	Acetaldehyde	60	30.36	0.2	3.7
4/6/2009	14	Acetic Acid	60	23.96	7	120
4/6/2009	15	Formaldehyde	60	30.04	5.1	140
4/6/2009	15	Acetaldehyde	60	30.04	0.2	3.7
4/6/2009	15	Acetic Acid	60	24.09	7	120
4/6/2009	16	Formaldehyde	60	30.13	ND	ND
4/6/2009	16	Acetic Acid	60	24.03	ND	ND
4/6/2009	17	Formaldehyde	NA	NA	ND	ND
4/6/2009	17	Acetic Acid	NA	NA	ND	ND
4/9/2009	1	Formaldehyde	60	30.67	18	480
4/9/2009	1	Acetaldehyde	60	30.67	0.2	3.6
4/9/2009	2	Formaldehyde	60	30.31	6.6	180
4/9/2009	2	Acetaldehyde	60	30.31	0.2	3.7
4/9/2009	4	Formaldehyde	60	30.76	8.4	220
4/9/2009	4	Acetaldehyde	60	30.76	0.2	3.6
4/9/2009	5	Formaldehyde	60	30.68	7.9	210
4/9/2009	6	Formaldehyde	60	30.31	10	270

Date	Trailer	Analyte	Sample Duration (minutes)	Sample Volume (liters)	Sample Mass (μg)	Concentration (ppb)
4/9/2009	6	Acetaldehyde	60	30.31	0.2	3.7
4/9/2009	7	Formaldehyde	60	30.58	8	210
4/9/2009	7	Acetaldehyde	60	30.58	0.3	5.4
4/9/2009	8	Formaldehyde	60	30.98	13	340
4/9/2009	9	Formaldehyde	60	30.23	2.2	59
4/9/2009	10	Formaldehyde	61	31.59	7.7	200
4/9/2009	10	Acetaldehyde	61	31.59	0.7	12
4/9/2009	11	Formaldehyde	60	30.14	14	380
4/9/2009	11	Acetaldehyde	60	30.14	0.5	9.2
4/9/2009	12	Formaldehyde	60	31.05	4.2	110
4/9/2009	12	Acetaldehyde	60	31.05	0.4	7.1
4/9/2009	13	Formaldehyde	60	30.65	4	110
4/9/2009	13	Acetaldehyde	60	30.65	0.5	9.1
4/9/2009	14	Formaldehyde	60	30.39	5.3	140
4/9/2009	14	Acetaldehyde	60	30.39	0.2	3.7
4/9/2009	15	Formaldehyde	60	30.60	6	160
4/9/2009	15	Acetaldehyde	60	30.60	0.3	5.4
4/9/2009	16	Formaldehyde	61	31.37	ND	ND
4/9/2009	17	Formaldehyde	NA	NA	ND	ND
4/13/2009	1	Formaldehyde	60	30.97	21	550
4/13/2009	1	Acetaldehyde	60	30.97	0.2	3.6
4/13/2009	1	Acetic Acid	60	24.50	15	250
4/13/2009	2	Formaldehyde	60	30.66	6.7	180
4/13/2009	2	Acetaldehyde	60	30.66	0.2	3.6
4/13/2009	2	Acetic Acid	60	24.07	12	200
4/13/2009	4	Formaldehyde	60	30.23	8.1	220
4/13/2009	4	Acetaldehyde	60	30.23	0.2	3.7
4/13/2009	4	Acetic Acid	60	24.14	13	220
4/13/2009	5	Formaldehyde	60	30.08	7.2	190
4/13/2009	5	Acetic Acid	60	24.12	12	200
4/13/2009	6	Formaldehyde	60	30.91	11	290
4/13/2009	6	Acetaldehyde	60	30.91	0.3	5.4
4/13/2009	6	Acetic Acid	60	24.05	11	190
4/13/2009	7	Formaldehyde	60	31.06	5.2	140
4/13/2009	7	Acetaldehyde	60	31.06	0.2	3.6
4/13/2009	7	Acetic Acid	60	24.55	6	100
4/13/2009	8	Formaldehyde	60	29.14	10	280
4/13/2009	8	Acetaldehyde	60	29.14	0.2	3.8
4/13/2009	8	Acetic Acid	60	24.43	13	220
4/13/2009	9	Formaldehyde	60	30.75	2.9	77
4/13/2009	9	Acetic Acid	60	24.18	2	34
4/13/2009	10	Formaldehyde	60	30.17	8.5	230
4/13/2009	10	Acetaldehyde	60	30.17	0.9	17
4/13/2009	10	Acetic Acid	60	24.45	6	100

Date	Trailer	Analyte	Sample Duration (minutes)	Sample Volume (liters)	Sample Mass (μg)	Concentration (ppb)
4/13/2009	11	Formaldehyde	60	30.17	13	350
4/13/2009	11	Acetaldehyde	60	30.17	0.5	9.2
4/13/2009	11	Acetic Acid	60	24.50	13	220
4/13/2009	12	Formaldehyde	60	30.58	4.4	120
4/13/2009	12	Acetaldehyde	60	30.58	0.4	7.3
4/13/2009	12	Acetic Acid	60	24.20	5	84
4/13/2009	13	Formaldehyde	60	30.72	4.1	110
4/13/2009	13	Acetaldehyde	60	30.72	0.6	11
4/13/2009	13	Acetic Acid	60	24.32	2	33
4/13/2009	14	Formaldehyde	60	31.34	5.4	140
4/13/2009	14	Acetaldehyde	60	31.34	0.2	3.5
4/13/2009	14	Acetic Acid	60	24.38	5	84
4/13/2009	15	Formaldehyde	60	30.08	6	160
4/13/2009	15	Acetaldehyde	60	30.08	0.3	5.5
4/13/2009	15	Acetic Acid	60	24.90	6	98
4/13/2009	16	Formaldehyde	60	30.97	ND	ND
4/13/2009	16	Acetic Acid	60	24.44	ND	ND
4/13/2009	17	Formaldehyde	NA	NA	ND	ND
4/13/2009	17	Acetic Acid	NA	NA	ND	ND
4/16/2009	1	Formaldehyde	60	31.33	18	470
4/16/2009	2	Formaldehyde	60	31.62	6.8	170
4/16/2009	2	Acetaldehyde	60	31.62	0.2	3.5
4/16/2009	4	Formaldehyde	60	30.43	8.5	230
4/16/2009	4	Acetaldehyde	60	30.43	0.2	3.6
4/16/2009	5	Formaldehyde	60	30.90	9	240
4/16/2009	6	Formaldehyde	60	31.25	12	310
4/16/2009	6	Acetaldehyde	60	31.25	0.3	5.3
4/16/2009	7	Formaldehyde	60	31.40	8.1	210
4/16/2009	7	Acetaldehyde	60	31.40	0.3	5.3
4/16/2009	8	Formaldehyde	60	30.89	13	340
4/16/2009	8	Acetaldehyde	60	30.89	0.3	5.4
4/16/2009	9	Formaldehyde	60	30.62	1.8	48
4/16/2009	10	Formaldehyde	60	30.87	8.7	230
4/16/2009	10	Acetaldehyde	60	30.87	0.7	13
4/16/2009	11	Formaldehyde	60	30.29	19	510
4/16/2009	11	Acetaldehyde	60	30.29	0.5	9.2
4/16/2009	12	Formaldehyde	60	30.88	4.8	130
4/16/2009	12	Acetaldehyde	60	30.88	0.4	7.2
4/16/2009	13	Formaldehyde	60	30.30	4.5	120
4/16/2009	13	Acetaldehyde	60	30.30	0.5	9.2
4/16/2009	14	Formaldehyde	60	31.17	5.9	150
4/16/2009	14	Acetaldehyde	60	31.17	0.3	5.3
4/16/2009	15	Formaldehyde	60	30.75	6.3	170
4/16/2009	15	Acetaldehyde	60	30.75	0.2	3.6

Date	Trailer	Analyte	Sample Duration (minutes)	Sample Volume (liters)	Sample Mass (μg)	Concentration (ppb)
4/16/2009	16	Formaldehyde	60	30.98	ND	ND
4/16/2009	17	Formaldehyde	NA	NA	ND	ND
5/4/2009	1	Formaldehyde	60	30.86	19	500
5/4/2009	1	Acetaldehyde	60	30.86	0.2	3.6
5/4/2009	1	Acetic Acid	60	23.99	13	220
5/4/2009	2	Formaldehyde	60	31.26	8.1	210
5/4/2009	2	Acetaldehyde	60	31.26	0.2	3.6
5/4/2009	2	Acetic Acid	60	24.63	10	170
5/4/2009	3	Formaldehyde	60	30.28	7.5	200
5/4/2009	3	Acetic Acid	60	24.35	6	100
5/4/2009	4	Formaldehyde	60	30.73	9.8	260
5/4/2009	4	Acetaldehyde	60	30.73	0.3	5.4
5/4/2009	4	Acetic Acid	60	24.32	10	170
5/4/2009	5	Formaldehyde	60	30.86	12	320
5/4/2009	5	Acetaldehyde	60	30.86	0.3	5.4
5/4/2009	5	Acetic Acid	60	24.21	12	200
5/4/2009	6	Formaldehyde	60	31.36	13	340
5/4/2009	6	Acetaldehyde	60	31.36	0.2	3.5
5/4/2009	6	Acetic Acid	60	24.40	9	150
5/4/2009	7	Formaldehyde	60	30.77	9.9	260
5/4/2009	7	Acetaldehyde	60	30.77	0.2	3.6
5/4/2009	7	Acetic Acid	60	24.38	9	150
5/4/2009	8	Formaldehyde	60	30.63	15	400
5/4/2009	8	Acetaldehyde	60	30.63	0.2	3.6
5/4/2009	8	Acetic Acid	60	24.51	11	180
5/4/2009	9	Formaldehyde	60	31.14	12	310
5/4/2009	9	Acetaldehyde	60	31.14	0.2	3.6
5/4/2009	9	Acetic Acid	60	24.70	7	120
5/4/2009	10	Formaldehyde	60	30.22	17	460
5/4/2009	10	Acetaldehyde	60	30.22	0.3	5.5
5/4/2009	10	Acetic Acid	60	24.85	12	200
5/4/2009	11	Formaldehyde	60	30.95	18	470
5/4/2009	11	Acetaldehyde	60	30.95	0.3	5.4
5/4/2009	11	Acetic Acid	60	24.51	11	180
5/4/2009	12	Formaldehyde	60	30.93	9.6	250
5/4/2009	12	Acetaldehyde	60	30.93	0.2	3.6
5/4/2009	12	Acetic Acid	60	24.38	8	130
5/4/2009	13	Formaldehyde	60	30.73	11	290
5/4/2009	13	Acetaldehyde	60	30.73	0.2	3.6
5/4/2009	13	Acetic Acid	60	24.64	8	130
5/4/2009	14	Formaldehyde	60	31.23	7.7	200
5/4/2009	14	Acetaldehyde	60	31.23	0.2	3.6
5/4/2009	14	Acetic Acid	60	24.53	8	130
5/4/2009	15	Formaldehyde	60	31.42	11	290

Date	Trailer	Analyte	Sample Duration (minutes)	Sample Volume (liters)	Sample Mass (μg)	Concentration (ppb)
5/4/2009	15	Acetaldehyde	60	31.42	0.4	7.1
5/4/2009	15	Acetic Acid	60	24.68	11	180
5/4/2009	16	Formaldehyde	60	31.26	ND	ND
5/4/2009	16	Acetic Acid	60	25.77	ND	ND
5/4/2009	17	Formaldehyde	NA	NA	ND	ND
5/4/2009	17	Acetic Acid	NA	NA	ND	ND
5/6/2009	1	Formaldehyde	60	31.36	15	390
5/6/2009	1	Acetaldehyde	60	31.36	0.2	3.5
5/6/2009	2	Formaldehyde	60	31.17	6.2	160
5/6/2009	2	Acetaldehyde	60	31.17	0.3	5.3
5/6/2009	3	Formaldehyde	60	31.65	6.5	170
5/6/2009	4	Formaldehyde	60	30.47	7.7	210
5/6/2009	4	Acetaldehyde	60	30.47	0.2	3.6
5/6/2009	5	Formaldehyde	60	30.41	10	270
5/6/2009	5	Acetaldehyde	60	30.41	0.3	5.5
5/6/2009	6	Formaldehyde	60	30.17	12	320
5/6/2009	6	Acetaldehyde	60	30.17	0.2	3.7
5/6/2009	7	Formaldehyde	60	30.74	8.7	230
5/6/2009	7	Acetaldehyde	60	30.74	0.2	3.6
5/6/2009	8	Formaldehyde	60	30.99	12	320
5/6/2009	8	Acetaldehyde	60	30.99	0.2	3.6
5/6/2009	9	Formaldehyde	60	31.14	11	290
5/6/2009	9	Acetaldehyde	60	31.14	0.3	5.3
5/6/2009	10	Formaldehyde	60	30.96	16	420
5/6/2009	10	Acetaldehyde	60	30.96	0.4	7.2
5/6/2009	11	Formaldehyde	60	30.68	14	370
5/6/2009	11	Acetaldehyde	60	30.68	0.3	5.4
5/6/2009	12	Formaldehyde	60	31.27	8.7	230
5/6/2009	12	Acetaldehyde	60	31.27	0.2	3.6
5/6/2009	13	Formaldehyde	60	30.39	8.8	240
5/6/2009	13	Acetaldehyde	60	30.39	0.2	3.7
5/6/2009	14	Formaldehyde	60	30.95	7.3	190
5/6/2009	14	Acetaldehyde	60	30.95	0.3	5.4
5/6/2009	15	Formaldehyde	60	30.62	9.4	250
5/6/2009	15	Acetaldehyde	60	30.62	0.4	7.3
5/6/2009	16	Formaldehyde	60	31.71	ND	ND
5/6/2009	17	Formaldehyde	NA	NA	ND	ND
5/8/2009	1	Formaldehyde	60	31.11	15	390
5/8/2009	1	Acetaldehyde	60	31.11	0.3	5.4
5/8/2009	1	Acetic Acid	60	24.24	5	84
5/8/2009	2	Formaldehyde	60	30.45	5.1	140
5/8/2009	2	Acetaldehyde	60	30.45	0.2	3.6
5/8/2009	2	Acetic Acid	60	24.87	5	82
5/8/2009	3	Formaldehyde	60	31.47	5.5	140

Date	Trailer	Analyte	Sample Duration (minutes)	Sample Volume (liters)	Sample Mass (μg)	Concentration (ppb)
5/8/2009	3	Acetic Acid	60	24.78	5	82
5/8/2009	4	Formaldehyde	60	31.22	6.4	170
5/8/2009	4	Acetaldehyde	60	31.22	0.3	5.3
5/8/2009	4	Acetic Acid	60	24.38	8	130
5/8/2009	5	Formaldehyde	60	30.79	6.3	170
5/8/2009	5	Acetaldehyde	60	30.79	0.2	3.6
5/8/2009	5	Acetic Acid	60	24.62	5	83
5/8/2009	6	Formaldehyde	60	30.59	8.6	230
5/8/2009	6	Acetaldehyde	60	30.59	0.2	3.6
5/8/2009	6	Acetic Acid	60	24.97	ND	ND
5/8/2009	7	Formaldehyde	60	32.06	7.1	180
5/8/2009	7	Acetaldehyde	60	32.06	0.2	3.5
5/8/2009	7	Acetic Acid	60	24.71	2	33
5/8/2009	8	Formaldehyde	60	30.96	11	290
5/8/2009	8	Acetaldehyde	60	30.96	0.2	3.6
5/8/2009	8	Acetic Acid	60	24.94	6	98
5/8/2009	9	Formaldehyde	60	31.34	7.6	200
5/8/2009	9	Acetaldehyde	60	31.34	0.2	3.5
5/8/2009	9	Acetic Acid	60	24.91	5	82
5/8/2009	10	Formaldehyde	60	31.06	12	310
5/8/2009	10	Acetaldehyde	60	31.06	0.3	5.4
5/8/2009	10	Acetic Acid	60	25.62	7	110
5/8/2009	11	Formaldehyde	60	31.13	13	340
5/8/2009	11	Acetaldehyde	60	31.13	0.3	5.3
5/8/2009	11	Acetic Acid	60	25.57	6	96
5/8/2009	12	Formaldehyde	60	31.38	6	160
5/8/2009	12	Acetic Acid	60	25.08	4	65
5/8/2009	13	Formaldehyde	60	30.71	7.5	200
5/8/2009	13	Acetic Acid	60	25.12	4	65
5/8/2009	14	Formaldehyde	60	31.14	4.3	110
5/8/2009	14	Acetic Acid	60	25.47	5	80
5/8/2009	15	Formaldehyde	60	31.35	7.1	180
5/8/2009	15	Acetaldehyde	60	31.35	0.3	5.3
5/8/2009	15	Acetic Acid	60	25.29	6	97
5/8/2009	16	Formaldehyde	60	30.50	ND	ND
5/8/2009	16	Acetic Acid	32	13.07	ND	ND
5/8/2009	17	Formaldehyde	NA	NA	ND	ND
5/8/2009	17	Acetic Acid	NA	NA	ND	ND
5/11/2009	1	Formaldehyde	60	32.95	15	370
5/11/2009	1	Acetaldehyde	60	32.95	0.3	5.1
5/11/2009	1	Acetic Acid	60	25.12	5	81
5/11/2009	2	Formaldehyde	60	30.69	4.2	110
5/11/2009	2	Acetaldehyde	60	30.69	0.3	5.4
5/11/2009	2	Acetic Acid	60	25.49	3	48

Date	Trailer	Analyte	Sample Duration (minutes)	Sample Volume (liters)	Sample Mass (µg)	Concentration (ppb)
5/11/2009	3	Formaldehyde	60	32.18	4.7	120
5/11/2009	3	Acetic Acid	60	24.63	2	33
5/11/2009	4	Formaldehyde	60	31.59	5.8	150
5/11/2009	4	Acetaldehyde	60	31.59	0.2	3.5
5/11/2009	4	Acetic Acid	60	24.86	5	82
5/11/2009	5	Formaldehyde	60	31.30	7.1	180
5/11/2009	5	Acetaldehyde	60	31.30	0.3	5.3
5/11/2009	5	Acetic Acid	60	25.47	3	48
5/11/2009	6	Formaldehyde	60	32.73	9.2	230
5/11/2009	6	Acetaldehyde	60	32.73	0.2	3.4
5/11/2009	6	Acetic Acid	60	24.99	2	33
5/11/2009	7	Formaldehyde	60	31.25	6.3	160
5/11/2009	7	Acetaldehyde	60	31.25	0.3	5.3
5/11/2009	7	Acetic Acid	60	25.30	3	48
5/11/2009	8	Formaldehyde	60	32.89	13	320
5/11/2009	8	Acetaldehyde	60	32.89	0.3	5.1
5/11/2009	8	Acetic Acid	60	24.71	4	66
5/11/2009	9	Formaldehyde	60	32.12	7.6	190
5/11/2009	9	Acetaldehyde	60	32.12	0.2	3.5
5/11/2009	9	Acetic Acid	60	25.24	4	65
5/11/2009	10	Formaldehyde	60	31.32	8.8	230
5/11/2009	10	Acetaldehyde	60	31.32	0.3	5.3
5/11/2009	10	Acetic Acid	60	24.86	5	82
5/11/2009	11	Formaldehyde	60	31.98	13	330
5/11/2009	11	Acetaldehyde	60	31.98	0.3	5.2
5/11/2009	11	Acetic Acid	60	25.41	5	80
5/11/2009	12	Formaldehyde	60	31.25	6.6	170
5/11/2009	12	Acetaldehyde	60	31.25	0.2	3.6
5/11/2009	12	Acetic Acid	60	24.43	ND	ND
5/11/2009	13	Formaldehyde	60	32.04	7.7	200
5/11/2009	13	Acetaldehyde	60	32.04	0.3	5.2
5/11/2009	13	Acetic Acid	60	25.37	2	32
5/11/2009	14	Formaldehyde	60	30.84	5.2	140
5/11/2009	14	Acetaldehyde	60	30.84	0.3	5.4
5/11/2009	14	Acetic Acid	60	25.56	2	32
5/11/2009	15	Formaldehyde	60	30.84	6.5	170
5/11/2009	15	Acetaldehyde	60	30.84	0.4	7.2
5/11/2009	15	Acetic Acid	60	26.05	4	63
5/11/2009	16	Formaldehyde	60	30.93	ND	ND
5/11/2009	16	Acetic Acid	60	26.06	ND	ND
5/11/2009	17	Formaldehyde	NA	NA	ND	ND
5/11/2009	17	Acetic Acid	NA	NA	ND	ND
5/13/2009	1	Formaldehyde	60	32.13	16	410
5/13/2009	1	Acetaldehyde	60	32.13	0.3	5.2

Date	Trailer	Analyte	Sample Duration (minutes)	Sample Volume (liters)	Sample Mass (μg)	Concentration (ppb)
5/13/2009	2	Formaldehyde	60	32.69	6.2	150
5/13/2009	2	Acetaldehyde	60	32.69	0.3	5.1
5/13/2009	3	Formaldehyde	60	30.88	5.5	150
5/13/2009	3	Acetaldehyde	60	30.88	0.2	3.6
5/13/2009	4	Formaldehyde	60	31.42	6.9	180
5/13/2009	4	Acetaldehyde	60	31.42	0.2	3.5
5/13/2009	5	Formaldehyde	60	30.77	9.2	240
5/13/2009	5	Acetaldehyde	60	30.77	0.3	5.4
5/13/2009	6	Formaldehyde	60	32.15	11	280
5/13/2009	6	Acetaldehyde	60	32.15	0.2	3.5
5/13/2009	7	Formaldehyde	60	31.79	8.1	210
5/13/2009	7	Acetaldehyde	60	31.79	0.3	5.2
5/13/2009	8	Formaldehyde	60	31.18	12	310
5/13/2009	8	Acetaldehyde	60	31.18	0.2	3.6
5/13/2009	9	Formaldehyde	60	31.47	10	260
5/13/2009	9	Acetaldehyde	60	31.47	0.3	5.3
5/13/2009	10	Formaldehyde	60	30.80	14	370
5/13/2009	10	Acetaldehyde	60	30.80	0.4	7.2
5/13/2009	11	Formaldehyde	60	31.58	14	360
5/13/2009	11	Acetaldehyde	60	31.58	0.3	5.3
5/13/2009	12	Formaldehyde	60	30.95	7.3	190
5/13/2009	12	Acetaldehyde	60	30.95	0.2	3.6
5/13/2009	13	Formaldehyde	60	30.51	8.7	230
5/13/2009	13	Acetaldehyde	60	30.51	0.4	7.3
5/13/2009	14	Formaldehyde	60	30.51	6.6	180
5/13/2009	15	Formaldehyde	60	30.82	8	210
5/13/2009	15	Acetaldehyde	60	30.82	0.2	3.6
5/13/2009	16	Formaldehyde	60	31.45	ND	ND
5/13/2009	17	Formaldehyde	NA	NA	ND	ND
5/15/2009	1	Formaldehyde	60	30.78	17	450
5/15/2009	1	Acetaldehyde	60	30.78	0.2	3.6
5/15/2009	1	Acetic Acid	60	25.50	7	110
5/15/2009	2	Formaldehyde	60	31.41	5.8	150
5/15/2009	2	Acetaldehyde	60	31.41	0.3	5.3
5/15/2009	2	Acetic Acid	60	25.27	5	81
5/15/2009	3	Formaldehyde	60	30.98	6	160
5/15/2009	3	Acetaldehyde	60	30.98	0.3	5.4
5/15/2009	3	Acetic Acid	60	25.57	4	64
5/15/2009	4	Formaldehyde	60	30.72	7	190
5/15/2009	4	Acetic Acid	60	25.42	5	80
5/15/2009	5	Formaldehyde	60	31.24	9.1	240
5/15/2009	5	Acetaldehyde	60	31.24	0.2	3.6
5/15/2009	5	Acetic Acid	60	25.11	3	49
5/15/2009	6	Formaldehyde	60	32.08	12	300

138

Date	Trailer	Analyte	Sample Duration (minutes)	Sample Volume (liters)	Sample Mass (μg)	Concentration (ppb)
5/15/2009	6	Acetaldehyde	60	32.08	0.2	3.5
5/15/2009	6	Acetic Acid	60	25.18	2	32
5/15/2009	7	Formaldehyde	60	31.51	7.2	190
5/15/2009	7	Acetaldehyde	60	31.51	0.3	5.3
5/15/2009	7	Acetic Acid	60	25.01	3	49
5/15/2009	8	Formaldehyde	60	31.21	12	310
5/15/2009	8	Acetaldehyde	60	31.21	0.2	3.6
5/15/2009	8	Acetic Acid	60	24.83	5	82
5/15/2009	9	Formaldehyde	60	31.83	11	280
5/15/2009	9	Acetaldehyde	60	31.83	0.2	3.5
5/15/2009	9	Acetic Acid	60	25.17	5	81
5/15/2009	10	Formaldehyde	60	31.75	14	360
5/15/2009	10	Acetaldehyde	60	31.75	0.3	5.2
5/15/2009	10	Acetic Acid	60	25.48	5	80
5/15/2009	11	Formaldehyde	60	30.71	15	400
5/15/2009	11	Acetaldehyde	60	30.71	0.3	5.4
5/15/2009	11	Acetic Acid	60	24.85	6	98
5/15/2009	12	Formaldehyde	60	31.59	7.7	200
5/15/2009	12	Acetaldehyde	60	31.59	0.4	7.0
5/15/2009	12	Acetic Acid	60	24.87	3	49
5/15/2009	13	Formaldehyde	60	31.35	9.3	240
5/15/2009	13	Acetaldehyde	60	31.35	0.2	3.5
5/15/2009	13	Acetic Acid	60	24.93	2	33
5/15/2009	14	Formaldehyde	60	31.09	6.8	180
5/15/2009	14	Acetaldehyde	60	31.09	0.3	5.4
5/15/2009	14	Acetic Acid	60	25.01	2	33
5/15/2009	15	Formaldehyde	60	30.58	8.6	230
5/15/2009	15	Acetaldehyde	60	30.58	0.4	7.3
5/15/2009	15	Acetic Acid	60	24.97	4	65
5/15/2009	16	Formaldehyde	60	30.71	ND	ND
5/15/2009	16	Acetic Acid	60	25.17	ND	ND
5/15/2009	17	Formaldehyde	NA	NA	ND	ND
5/15/2009	17	Acetic Acid	NA	NA	ND	ND

Volatile Organic Compound (VOC) air sample results. Results are provided for those compounds identified or tentatively identified (qualifier J). Note: Trailer 16 is an ambient sample, 17 is a field blank, and 18 is a media blank. NA–Not applicable.

Date	Trailer	Analyte	Sample Duration (minutes)	Sample Volume (liters)	Sample Mass (μg)	Concentration (ppb)	Qual-ifier
12/16/2008	1	2-butanone (MEK)	61	6.05	0.058	3.3	
12/16/2008	1	4-methyl-2-pentanone	61	6.05	0.056	2.3	
12/16/2008	1	acetic acid	61	6.05	6.3	420	J
12/16/2008	1	dibutyl phthalate	61	6.05	0.14	2.0	J
12/16/2008	1	formic acid	61	6.05	0.35	31	J
12/16/2008	1	Freon 113	61	6.05	0.027	0.90	
12/16/2008	1	methylene chloride	61	6.05	0.14	6.7	
12/16/2008	2	acetic acid	61	5.94	0.9	62	J
12/16/2008	2	α-pinene	61	5.94	0.13	3.9	J
12/16/2008	2	dibutyl phthalate	61	5.94	0.23	3.4	J
12/16/2008	2	methylene chloride	61	5.94	0.069	3.4	
12/16/2008	2	nonanal	61	5.94	0.11	3.2	J
12/16/2008	2	propanoic acid, 2-methyl	61	5.94	0.064	3.6	J
12/16/2008	2	styrene	61	5.94	0.028	1.1	
12/16/2008	2	tetradecane	61	5.94	0.058	1.2	J
12/16/2008	2	triacetin	61	5.94	0.045	0.85	J
12/16/2008	3	acetic acid	61	5.95	1.4	96	J
12/16/2008	3	acetone	61	5.95	0.042	3.0	
12/16/2008	3	α-pinene	61	5.95	0.14	4.2	J
12/16/2008	3	dibutyl phthalate	61	5.95	2.5	37	J
12/16/2008	3	methylene chloride	61	5.95	0.057	2.8	
12/16/2008	3	nonanal	61	5.95	0.12	3.5	J
12/16/2008	3	triacetin	61	5.95	0.11	2.1	J
12/16/2008	3	tridecane	61	5.95	0.11	2.5	J
12/16/2008	4	acetic acid	61	6.52	1.2	75	J
12/16/2008	4	α-pinene	61	6.52	0.19	5.2	J
12/16/2008	4	C7 alkene	61	6.52	0.08	3.1	J
12/16/2008	4	dibutyl phthalate	61	6.52	2.8	38	J
12/16/2008	4	formic acid	61	6.52	0.1	8.2	J
12/16/2008	4	methylene chloride	61	6.52	0.043	1.9	
12/16/2008	4	nonanal	61	6.52	0.095	2.5	J
12/16/2008	4	tetradecane	61	6.52	0.081	1.5	J
12/16/2008	4	tridecane	61	6.52	0.086	1.8	J
12/16/2008	5	4-methyl-2-pentanone	62	6.26	0.03	1.2	
12/16/2008	5	acetic acid	62	6.26	1.7	110	J
12/16/2008	5	α-pinene	62	6.26	0.17	4.9	J
12/16/2008	5	dibutyl phthalate	62	6.26	2.1	29	J
12/16/2008	5	formic acid	62	6.26	0.11	9.3	J
12/16/2008	5	hexanal	62	6.26	0.086	3.3	J

Date	Trailer	Analyte	Sample Duration (minutes)	Sample Volume (liters)	Sample Mass (μg)	Concen-tration (ppb)	Qual-ifier
12/16/2008	5	methylene chloride	62	6.26	0.032	1.5	
12/16/2008	5	nonanal	62	6.26	0.1	2.8	J
12/16/2008	5	styrene	62	6.26	0.025	0.94	
12/16/2008	5	tetradecane	62	6.26	0.069	1.4	J
12/16/2008	5	toluene	62	6.26	0.029	1.2	
12/16/2008	6	acetic acid	61	6.13	0.076	5.1	J
12/16/2008	6	α-pinene	61	6.13	0.099	2.9	J
12/16/2008	6	C7 alkene	61	6.13	0.057	2.3	J
12/16/2008	6	dibutyl phthalate	61	6.13	2.2	32	J
12/16/2008	6	hexanal	61	6.13	0.068	2.7	J
12/16/2008	6	methylene chloride	61	6.13	0.027	1.3	
12/16/2008	6	nonanal	61	6.13	0.11	3.1	J
12/16/2008	6	tetradecane	61	6.13	0.081	1.6	J
12/16/2008	7	2-butanone (MEK)	62	6.43	0.025	1.3	
12/16/2008	7	acetic acid	62	6.43	0.94	60	J
12/16/2008	7	α-pinene	62	6.43	0.22	6.1	J
12/16/2008	7	C7 alkene	62	6.43	0.072	2.8	J
12/16/2008	7	dibutyl phthalate	62	6.43	2.3	31	J
12/16/2008	7	hexanal	62	6.43	0.06	2.2	J
12/16/2008	7	nonanal	62	6.43	0.069	1.8	J
12/16/2008	7	tetradecane	62	6.43	0.098	1.9	J
12/16/2008	7	tridecane	62	6.43	0.067	1.4	J
12/16/2008	8	4-methyl-2-pentanone	60	6.01	0.029	1.2	
12/16/2008	8	acetic acid	60	6.01	2.2	150	J
12/16/2008	8	acetone	60	6.01	0.045	3.2	
12/16/2008	8	α-pinene	60	6.01	0.18	5.4	J
12/16/2008	8	dibutyl phthalate	60	6.01	0.65	9.5	J
12/16/2008	8	dichlorodifluormethane	60	6.01	0.036	1.2	
12/16/2008	8	formic acid	60	6.01	0.1	8.8	J
12/16/2008	8	hexanal	60	6.01	0.073	2.9	J
12/16/2008	8	nonanal	60	6.01	0.089	2.5	J
12/16/2008	8	pentanal	60	6.01	0.026	1.2	J
12/16/2008	8	phenol	60	6.01	0.071	3.1	J
12/16/2008	8	tetradecane	60	6.01	0.091	1.9	J
12/16/2008	8	toluene	60	6.01	0.029	1.3	
12/16/2008	9	acetic acid	60	5.97	1.6	89	J
12/16/2008	9	α-pinene	60	5.97	0.18	5.4	J
12/16/2008	9	dibutyl phthalate	60	5.97	1.5	22	J
12/16/2008	9	formic acid	60	5.97	0.088	7.8	J
12/16/2008	9	hexanal	60	5.97	0.056	2.3	J
12/16/2008	9	nonanal	60	5.97	0.078	2.3	J
12/16/2008	9	tetradecane	60	5.97	0.063	1.3	J

Date	Trailer	Analyte	Sample Duration (minutes)	Sample Volume (liters)	Sample Mass (μg)	Concen-tration (ppb)	Qual-ifier
12/16/2008	9	triacetin	60	5.97	0.039	0.73	J
12/16/2008	9	tridecane	60	5.97	0.036	0.80	J
12/16/2008	10	2-butanone (MEK)	60	6.00	0.032	1.8	
12/16/2008	10	toluene	60	6.00	0.028	1.2	
12/16/2008	11	4-methyl-2-pentanone	64	6.46	0.04	1.5	
12/16/2008	11	acetic acid	64	6.46	1.3	82	J
12/16/2008	11	α-pinene	64	6.46	0.2	5.6	J
12/16/2008	11	dibutyl phthalate	64	6.46	0.81	11	J
12/16/2008	11	formic acid	64	6.46	0.15	12	J
12/16/2008	11	hexanal	64	6.46	0.097	3.6	J
12/16/2008	11	nonanal	64	6.46	0.095	2.5	J
12/16/2008	11	tetradecane	64	6.46	0.067	1.3	J
12/16/2008	12	acetic acid	66	6.60	2.1	130	J
12/16/2008	12	acetone	66	6.60	0.052	3.3	
12/16/2008	12	α-pinene	66	6.60	0.17	4.6	J
12/16/2008	12	C7 alkene	66	6.60	0.06	2.3	J
12/16/2008	12	dibutyl phthalate	66	6.60	0.43	5.7	J
12/16/2008	12	dichlorodifluormethane	66	6.60	0.035	1.1	
12/16/2008	12	ethanol	66	6.60	0.058	4.7	
12/16/2008	12	formic acid	66	6.60	0.063	5.1	J
12/16/2008	12	hexanal	66	6.60	0.065	2.4	J
12/16/2008	12	methylene chloride	66	6.60	0.029	1.3	
12/16/2008	12	nonanal	66	6.60	0.11	2.9	J
12/16/2008	12	phenol	66	6.60	0.096	3.8	J
12/16/2008	12	propanoic acid, 2-methyl	66	6.60	0.095	4.0	J
12/16/2008	13	acetic acid	65	6.51	1.6	100	J
12/16/2008	13	α-pinene	65	6.51	0.22	6.1	J
12/16/2008	13	C7 alkene	65	6.51	0.067	2.6	J
12/16/2008	13	dibutyl phthalate	65	6.51	1.1	15	J
12/16/2008	13	formic acid	65	6.51	0.24	20	J
12/16/2008	13	hexanal	65	6.51	0.062	2.3	J
12/16/2008	13	isopropyl alcohol	65	6.51	0.078	4.9	
12/16/2008	13	nonanal	65	6.51	0.075	2.0	J
12/16/2008	14	acetic acid	68	6.76	0.61	37	J
12/16/2008	14	α-pinene	68	6.76	0.15	4.0	J
12/16/2008	14	dibutyl phthalate	68	6.76	1.7	22	J
12/16/2008	14	formic acid	68	6.76	0.1	7.9	J
12/16/2008	14	hexanal	68	6.76	0.04	1.4	J
12/16/2008	14	nonanal	68	6.76	0.088	2.2	J
12/16/2008	14	tetradecane	68	6.76	0.11	2.0	J
12/16/2008	16	dibutyl phthalate	60	6.01	1.2	18	J
12/16/2008	16	triacetin	60	6.01	0.015	0.28	J

Date	Trailer	Analyte	Sample Duration (minutes)	Sample Volume (liters)	Sample Mass (μg)	Concen-tration (ppb)	Qual-ifier
12/16/2008	17	acetic acid	0	0	0.017	N/A	J
12/16/2008	17	butane, 2-methyl-	0	0	0.025	N/A	J
12/16/2008	17	dibutyl phthalate	0	0	0.42	N/A	J
12/16/2008	17	triacetin	0	0	0.022	N/A	J
12/19/2008	1	acetone	68	7.27	0.05	2.9	
12/19/2008	1	α-pinene	68	7.27	0.23	19	J
12/19/2008	1	hexanal	68	7.27	0.17	5.6	J
12/19/2008	1	nonanal	68	7.27	0.14	5.6	J
12/19/2008	1	phenol	68	7.27	0.13	4.7	J
12/19/2008	1	tetradecane	68	7.27	0.12	2.0	J
12/19/2008	1	toluene	68	7.27	0.032	1.2	
12/19/2008	1	tridecane	68	7.27	0.044	0.80	J
12/19/2008	2	acetone	70	7.33	0.071	4.1	
12/19/2008	2	α-pinene	70	7.33	0.22	5.4	J
12/19/2008	2	formic acid	70	7.33	0.1	7.3	J
12/19/2008	2	hexanal	70	7.33	0.12	3.9	J
12/19/2008	2	nonanal	70	7.33	0.17	4.0	J
12/19/2008	2	phenol	70	7.33	0.097	3.4	J
12/19/2008	2	styrene	70	7.33	0.05	1.6	
12/19/2008	2	tetradecane	70	7.33	0.099	1.7	J
12/19/2008	2	tridecane	70	7.33	0.045	0.81	J
12/19/2008	3	acetic acid	71	7.13	0.99	57	J
12/19/2008	3	acetone	71	7.13	0.04	2.4	
12/19/2008	3	α-pinene	71	7.13	0.17	4.3	J
12/19/2008	3	formic acid	71	7.13	0.051	3.8	J
12/19/2008	3	hexanal	71	7.13	0.091	3.1	J
12/19/2008	3	nonanal	71	7.13	0.11	2.7	J
12/19/2008	3	phenol	71	7.13	0.076	2.8	J
12/19/2008	3	propanoic acid, 2-methyl	71	7.13	0.058	2.3	J
12/19/2008	3	tetradecane	71	7.13	0.086	1.5	J
12/19/2008	4	acetone	68	6.89	0.045	2.8	
12/19/2008	4	α-pinene	68	6.89	0.28	7.3	J
12/19/2008	4	formic acid	68	6.89	0.18	14	J
12/19/2008	4	hexanal	68	6.89	0.1	3.5	J
12/19/2008	4	phenol	68	6.89	0.094	3.5	J
12/19/2008	4	tetradecane	68	6.89	0.094	1.7	J
12/19/2008	4	tridecane	68	6.89	0.037	0.71	J
12/19/2008	5	4-methyl-2-pentanone	70	7.07	0.068	2.4	
12/19/2008	5	acetone	70	7.07	0.2	12	
12/19/2008	5	α-pinene	70	7.07	0.34	8.6	J
12/19/2008	5	dichlorodifluormethane	70	7.07	0.037	1.1	
12/19/2008	5	ethanol	70	7.07	0.062	4.7	

Date	Trailer	Analyte	Sample Duration (minutes)	Sample Volume (liters)	Sample Mass (μg)	Concentration (ppb)	Qual-ifier
12/19/2008	5	hexanal	70	7.07	0.15	5.1	J
12/19/2008	5	isopropyl alcohol	70	7.07	0.046	2.7	
12/19/2008	5	methylene chloride	70	7.07	0.2	8.1	
12/19/2008	5	nonanal	70	7.07	0.15	3.7	J
12/19/2008	5	phenol	70	7.07	0.12	4.4	J
12/19/2008	5	styrene	70	7.07	0.034	1.1	
12/19/2008	5	tetradecane	70	7.07	0.088	1.5	J
12/19/2008	5	toluene	70	7.07	0.049	1.8	
12/19/2008	5	tridecane	70	7.07	0.04	0.75	J
12/19/2008	6	acetone	71	7.14	0.049	2.9	
12/19/2008	6	α-pinene	71	7.14	0.18	4.5	J
12/19/2008	6	ethanol	71	7.14	0.031	2.3	
12/19/2008	6	hexanal	71	7.14	0.11	3.7	J
12/19/2008	6	methylene chloride	71	7.14	0.1	4.0	
12/19/2008	6	nonanal	71	7.14	0.12	2.9	J
12/19/2008	6	phenol	71	7.14	0.089	3.2	J
12/19/2008	6	tetradecane	71	7.14	0.096	1.7	J
12/19/2008	7	acetaldehyde	71	7.04	0.059	4.7	J
12/19/2008	7	acetone	71	7.04	0.066	4.0	
12/19/2008	7	α-pinene	71	7.04	0.26	6.6	J
12/19/2008	7	dichlorodifluormethane	71	7.04	0.032	0.92	
12/19/2008	7	hexanal	71	7.04	0.1	3.4	J
12/19/2008	7	methylene chloride	71	7.04	0.081	3.3	
12/19/2008	7	nonanal	71	7.04	0.082	2.0	J
12/19/2008	7	phenol	71	7.04	0.11	4.1	J
12/19/2008	7	styrene	71	7.04	0.037	1.2	
12/19/2008	7	tetradecane	71	7.04	0.12	2.1	J
12/19/2008	7	toluene	71	7.04	0.04	1.5	
12/19/2008	7	tridecane	71	7.04	0.058	1.1	J
12/19/2008	7	xylene	71	7.04	0.03	0.98	
12/19/2008	8	4-methyl-2-pentanone	65	6.53	0.064	2.4	
12/19/2008	8	acetone	65	6.53	0.048	3.1	
12/19/2008	8	α-pinene	65	6.53	0.25	6.9	J
12/19/2008	8	formic acid	65	6.53	0.24	20	J
12/19/2008	8	hexanal	65	6.53	0.14	5.1	J
12/19/2008	8	methylene chloride	65	6.53	0.093	4.1	
12/19/2008	8	nonanal	65	6.53	0.13	3.4	J
12/19/2008	8	phenol	65	6.53	0.13	5.2	J
12/19/2008	8	styrene	65	6.53	0.05	1.8	
12/19/2008	8	tetradecane	65	6.53	0.12	2.3	J
12/19/2008	8	toluene	65	6.53	0.06	2.4	
12/19/2008	8	tridecane	65	6.53	0.039	0.79	J

Date	Trailer	Analyte	Sample Duration (minutes)	Sample Volume (liters)	Sample Mass (μg)	Concentration (ppb)	Qual-ifier
12/19/2008	8	xylene	65	6.53	0.026	0.92	
12/19/2008	9	acetic acid	63	6.36	1.4	90	J
12/19/2008	9	acetone	63	6.36	0.063	4.2	
12/19/2008	9	α-pinene	63	6.36	0.29	8.2	J
12/19/2008	9	dichlorodifluormethane	63	6.36	0.04	1.3	
12/19/2008	9	ethanol	63	6.36	0.057	4.8	
12/19/2008	9	formic acid	63	6.36	0.059	4.9	J
12/19/2008	9	hexanal	63	6.36	0.11	4.1	J
12/19/2008	9	methylene chloride	63	6.36	0.053	2.8	
12/19/2008	9	nonanal	63	6.36	0.13	3.5	J
12/19/2008	9	phenol	63	6.36	0.087	3.6	J
12/19/2008	9	propanoic acid, 2-methyl	63	6.36	0.065	2.8	J
12/19/2008	9	tetradecane	63	6.36	0.099	1.9	J
12/19/2008	10	4-methyl-2-pentanone	61	6.18	0.087	3.4	
12/19/2008	10	acetic acid	61	6.18	2.9	190	J
12/19/2008	10	acetone	61	6.18	0.079	5.4	
12/19/2008	10	α-pinene	61	6.18	0.31	9.0	J
12/19/2008	10	ethanol	61	6.18	0.063	5.4	
12/19/2008	10	formic acid	61	6.18	0.21	18	J
12/19/2008	10	hexanal	61	6.18	0.17	6.6	J
12/19/2008	10	methylene chloride	61	6.18	0.067	3.1	
12/19/2008	10	nonanal	61	6.18	0.14	3.9	J
12/19/2008	10	phenol	61	6.18	0.095	4.0	J
12/19/2008	10	propanoic acid, 2-methyl	61	6.18	0.1	4.5	J
12/19/2008	10	tetradecane	61	6.18	0.069	1.4	J
12/19/2008	10	toluene	61	6.18	0.054	2.3	
12/19/2008	11	4-methyl-2-pentanone	60	6.03	0.099	4.0	
12/19/2008	11	acetic acid	60	6.03	1.8	120	J
12/19/2008	11	acetone	60	6.03	0.13	9.1	
12/19/2008	11	α-pinene	60	6.03	0.31	9.2	J
12/19/2008	11	dichlorodifluormethane	60	6.03	0.047	1.6	
12/19/2008	11	ethanol	60	6.03	0.063	5.6	
12/19/2008	11	formic acid	60	6.03	0.068	6.0	J
12/19/2008	11	hexanal	60	6.03	0.14	5.6	J
12/19/2008	11	methylene chloride	60	6.03	0.057	2.7	
12/19/2008	11	nonanal	60	6.03	0.12	3.4	J
12/19/2008	11	phenol	60	6.03	0.071	3.1	J
12/19/2008	11	propanoic acid, 2-methyl	60	6.03	0.06	2.8	J
12/19/2008	11	styrene	60	6.03	0.025	0.97	
12/19/2008	11	tetradecane	60	6.03	0.071	1.5	J
12/19/2008	11	toluene	60	6.03	0.026	1.1	
12/19/2008	12	acetic acid	60	6.06	1.4	94	J

Date	Trailer	Analyte	Sample Duration (minutes)	Sample Volume (liters)	Sample Mass (µg)	Concen- tration (ppb)	Qual -ifier
12/19/2008	12	acetone	60	6.06	0.089	6.2	
12/19/2008	12	α-pinene	60	6.06	0.2	5.9	J
12/19/2008	12	dichlorodifluormethane	60	6.06	0.049	1.6	
12/19/2008	12	ethanol	60	6.06	0.064	5.6	
12/19/2008	12	formic acid	60	6.06	0.06	5.3	J
12/19/2008	12	hexanal	60	6.06	0.1	4.0	J
12/19/2008	12	methylene chloride	60	6.06	0.054	2.6	
12/19/2008	12	nonanal	60	6.06	0.14	4.0	J
12/19/2008	12	phenol	60	6.06	0.091	3.9	J
12/19/2008	12	propanoic acid, 2-methyl	60	6.06	0.097	4.4	J
12/19/2008	12	styrene	60	6.06	0.027	1.1	
12/19/2008	12	tetradecane	60	6.06	0.1	2.0	J
12/19/2008	13	4-methyl-2-pentanone	60	6.31	0.031	1.2	
12/19/2008	13	acetic acid	60	6.31	1.1	71	J
12/19/2008	13	acetone	60	6.31	0.044	2.9	
12/19/2008	13	α-pinene	60	6.31	0.3	8.5	J
12/19/2008	13	formic acid	60	6.31	0.066	5.6	J
12/19/2008	13	hexanal	60	6.31	0.1	3.8	J
12/19/2008	13	nonanal	60	6.31	0.11	3.0	J
12/19/2008	13	phenol	60	6.31	0.072	3.0	J
12/19/2008	13	propanoic acid, 2-methyl	60	6.31	0.089	3.9	J
12/19/2008	13	tetradecane	60	6.31	0.09	1.8	J
12/19/2008	13	toluene	60	6.31	0.031	1.3	
12/19/2008	14	acetic acid	60	6.31	0.96	65	J
12/19/2008	14	acetone	60	6.31	0.034	2.4	
12/19/2008	14	α-pinene	60	6.31	0.24	7.1	J
12/19/2008	14	hexanal	60	6.31	0.073	2.9	J
12/19/2008	14	methylene chloride	60	6.31	0.031	1.5	
12/19/2008	14	nonanal	60	6.31	0.072	2.1	J
12/19/2008	14	phenol	60	6.31	0.065	2.8	J
12/19/2008	14	propanoic acid, 2-methyl	60	6.31	0.098	4.5	J
12/19/2008	14	tetradecane	60	6.31	0.065	1.3	J
12/19/2008	14	tridecane	60	6.31	0.09	2.0	J
12/19/2008	15	2-butanone (MEK)	60	6.02	0.028	1.6	
12/19/2008	15	4-methyl-2-pentanone	60	6.02	0.1	4.1	
12/19/2008	15	acetone	60	6.02	0.15	10	
12/19/2008	15	α-pinene	60	6.02	0.46	14	J
12/19/2008	15	dichlorodifluormethane	60	6.02	0.032	1.1	
12/19/2008	15	formic acid	60	6.02	0.1	8.8	J
12/19/2008	15	hexanal	60	6.02	0.19	7.6	J
12/19/2008	15	nonanal	60	6.02	0.14	4.0	J
12/19/2008	15	phenol	60	6.02	0.095	4.1	J

Date	Trailer	Analyte	Sample Duration (minutes)	Sample Volume (liters)	Sample Mass (µg)	Concen-tration (ppb)	Qual-ifier
12/19/2008	15	styrene	60	6.02	0.1	3.9	
12/19/2008	15	tetradecane	60	6.02	0.086	1.8	J
12/19/2008	15	toluene	60	6.02	0.066	2.9	
12/19/2008	16	acetaldehyde	60	6.05	0.03	2.8	
12/19/2008	16	acetic acid	60	6.05	0.026	1.8	J
12/19/2008	16	dichlorodifluormethane	60	6.05	0.031	1.0	
12/19/2008	17	acetic acid	0	0	0.019	N/A	J
1/16/2009	1	acetic acid	60	6.00	1.1	75	J
1/16/2009	1	acetone	60	6.00	0.083	5.8	
1/16/2009	1	α-pinene	60	6.00	0.043	1.3	J
1/16/2009	1	hexanal	60	6.00	0.022	0.88	J
1/16/2009	1	nonanal	60	6.00	0.044	2.1	J
1/16/2009	1	tetradecane	60	6.00	0.024	0.49	J
1/16/2009	2	acetic acid	60	6.00	0.24	16	J
1/16/2009	2	acetone	60	6.00	0.053	3.7	
1/16/2009	2	α-pinene	60	6.00	0.048	1.4	J
1/16/2009	2	dichlorodifluormethane	60	6.00	0.034	1.2	
1/16/2009	2	hexanal	60	6.00	0.021	0.84	J
1/16/2009	2	nonanal	60	6.00	0.045	1.3	J
1/16/2009	2	tetradecane	60	6.00	0.017	0.35	J
1/16/2009	3	acetic acid	60	6.00	0.084	5.7	J
1/16/2009	3	acetone	60	6.00	0.041	2.9	
1/16/2009	3	α-pinene	60	6.00	0.041	1.2	J
1/16/2009	3	dichlorodifluormethane	60	6.00	0.031	1.1	
1/16/2009	3	nonanal	60	6.00	0.028	0.80	J
1/16/2009	3	tetradecane	60	6.00	0.018	0.37	J
1/16/2009	4	acetic acid	60	6.04	0.2	13	J
1/16/2009	4	acetone	60	6.04	0.049	3.4	
1/16/2009	4	α-pinene	60	6.04	0.067	2.0	J
1/16/2009	4	dichlorodifluormethane	60	6.04	0.036	1.2	
1/16/2009	4	hexanal	60	6.04	0.021	0.83	J
1/16/2009	4	nonanal	60	6.04	0.024	0.68	J
1/16/2009	4	propanoic acid, 2-methyl	60	6.04	0.018	0.83	J
1/16/2009	4	tetradecane	60	6.04	0.022	0.45	J
1/16/2009	5	acetic acid	60	6.02	0.95	64	J
1/16/2009	5	acetone	60	6.02	0.059	4.1	
1/16/2009	5	α-pinene	60	6.02	0.078	2.3	J
1/16/2009	5	hexanal	60	6.02	0.024	0.95	J
1/16/2009	5	nonanal	60	6.02	0.042	1.2	J
1/16/2009	5	tetradecane	60	6.02	0.016	0.33	J
1/16/2009	6	acetic acid	60	6.03	0.12	8.1	J
1/16/2009	6	acetone	60	6.03	0.032	2.2	

Date	Trailer	Analyte	Sample Duration (minutes)	Sample Volume (liters)	Sample Mass (μg)	Concen-tration (ppb)	Qual-ifier
1/16/2009	6	α-pinene	60	6.03	0.037	1.1	J
1/16/2009	6	dichlorodifluormethane	60	6.03	0.037	1.2	
1/16/2009	6	hexanal	60	6.03	0.017	0.67	J
1/16/2009	6	nonanal	60	6.03	0.025	0.71	J
1/16/2009	6	tetradecane	60	6.03	0.016	0.33	J
1/16/2009	7	acetic acid	60	6.05	0.24	16	J
1/16/2009	7	acetone	60	6.05	0.056	3.9	
1/16/2009	7	α-pinene	60	6.05	0.065	1.9	J
1/16/2009	7	dichlorodifluormethane	60	6.05	0.028	0.94	
1/16/2009	7	hexanal	60	6.05	0.017	0.67	J
1/16/2009	7	nonanal	60	6.05	0.029	0.82	J
1/16/2009	7	tetradecane	60	6.05	0.029	0.59	J
1/16/2009	8	2-butanone (MEK)	60	6.00	0.026	1.5	
1/16/2009	8	acetic acid	60	6.00	0.26	18	J
1/16/2009	8	acetone	60	6.00	0.044	3.1	
1/16/2009	8	α-pinene	60	6.00	0.053	1.6	J
1/16/2009	8	dichlorodifluormethane	60	6.00	0.036	1.2	
1/16/2009	8	hexanal	60	6.00	0.022	0.88	J
1/16/2009	8	nonanal	60	6.00	0.037	1.1	J
1/16/2009	8	tetradecane	60	6.00	0.036	0.74	J
1/16/2009	9	2-butanone (MEK)	60	6.01	0.027	1.5	
1/16/2009	9	acetic acid	60	6.01	0.22	15	J
1/16/2009	9	acetone	60	6.01	0.059	4.1	
1/16/2009	9	α-pinene	60	6.01	0.067	2.0	J
1/16/2009	9	dichlorodifluormethane	60	6.01	0.036	1.2	
1/16/2009	9	hexanal	60	6.01	0.018	0.72	J
1/16/2009	9	nonanal	60	6.01	0.032	0.92	J
1/16/2009	9	tetradecane	60	6.01	0.02	0.41	J
1/16/2009	10	acetic acid	60	6.04	0.38	26	J
1/16/2009	10	acetone	60	6.04	0.038	2.7	
1/16/2009	10	α-pinene	60	6.04	0.072	2.1	J
1/16/2009	10	dichlorodifluormethane	60	6.04	0.032	1.1	
1/16/2009	10	hexanal	60	6.04	0.027	1.1	J
1/16/2009	10	nonanal	60	6.04	0.033	0.94	J
1/16/2009	11	acetaldehyde	60	6.02	0.031	2.9	J
1/16/2009	11	acetic acid	60	6.02	0.08	5.4	J
1/16/2009	11	acetonitrile	60	6.02	0.29	28.7	J
1/16/2009	11	butane, 2-methyl-	60	6.02	0.09	5.1	J
1/16/2009	11	dichlorodifluormethane	60	6.02	0.042	1.4	
1/16/2009	12	2-butanone (MEK)	60	5.99	0.039	2.2	
1/16/2009	12	acetic acid	60	5.99	0.14	9.5	J
1/16/2009	12	acetone	60	5.99	0.036	2.5	

Date	Trailer	Analyte	Sample Duration (minutes)	Sample Volume (liters)	Sample Mass (µg)	Concen-tration (ppb)	Qual-ifier
1/16/2009	12	α-pinene	60	5.99	0.05	1.5	J
1/16/2009	12	dichlorodifluormethane	60	5.99	0.057	1.9	
1/16/2009	12	hexanal	60	5.99	0.021	0.84	J
1/16/2009	12	nonanal	60	5.99	0.035	1.0	J
1/16/2009	12	tetradecane	60	5.99	0.018	0.37	J
1/16/2009	13	2-butanone (MEK)	60	6.02	0.037	2.1	
1/16/2009	13	acetic acid	60	6.02	0.15	10	J
1/16/2009	13	acetone	60	6.02	0.043	3.0	
1/16/2009	13	α-pinene	60	6.02	0.1	3.0	J
1/16/2009	13	dichlorodifluormethane	60	6.02	0.034	1.1	
1/16/2009	13	hexanal	60	6.02	0.02	0.79	J
1/16/2009	13	nonanal	60	6.02	0.036	1.0	J
1/16/2009	13	tetradecane	60	6.02	0.015	0.31	J
1/16/2009	13	toluene	60	6.02	0.032	1.4	
1/16/2009	14	2-butanone (MEK)	60	5.99	0.034	1.9	
1/16/2009	14	acetic acid	60	5.99	0.2	14	J
1/16/2009	14	acetone	60	5.99	0.072	5.1	
1/16/2009	14	α-pinene	60	5.99	0.059	1.8	J
1/16/2009	14	dichlorodifluormethane	60	5.99	0.036	1.2	
1/16/2009	14	nonanal	60	5.99	0.022	0.63	J
1/16/2009	14	tetradecane	60	5.99	0.024	0.49	J
1/16/2009	14	toluene	60	5.99	0.034	1.5	
1/16/2009	15	2-butanone (MEK)	60	6.05	0.03	1.7	
1/16/2009	15	acetic acid	60	6.05	0.31	21	J
1/16/2009	15	acetone	60	6.05	0.025	1.7	
1/16/2009	15	α-pinene	60	6.05	0.072	2.1	J
1/16/2009	15	hexanal	60	6.05	0.02	0.79	J
1/16/2009	15	nonanal	60	6.05	0.025	0.71	J
1/16/2009	15	toluene	60	6.05	0.025	1.1	
1/16/2009	16	2-butanone (MEK)	60	6.03	0.045	2.5	
1/16/2009	16	acetic acid	60	6.03	0.37	25	J
1/16/2009	16	acetone	60	6.03	0.038	2.7	
1/16/2009	16	α-pinene	60	6.03	0.08	2.4	J
1/16/2009	16	dichlorodifluormethane	60	6.03	0.054	1.8	
1/16/2009	16	hexanal	60	6.03	0.024	0.95	J
1/16/2009	16	nonanal	60	6.03	0.032	0.91	J
1/16/2009	16	tetradecane	60	6.03	0.018	0.37	J
1/16/2009	16	toluene	60	6.03	0.033	1.5	
1/16/2009	17	2-butanone (MEK)	0	0	0.035	N/A	
1/16/2009	17	acetaldehyde	0	0	0.038	N/A	J
1/16/2009	17	acetic acid	0	0	0.087	N/A	J
1/16/2009	17	acetone	0	0	0.051	N/A	

Date	Trailer	Analyte	Sample Duration (minutes)	Sample Volume (liters)	Sample Mass (μg)	Concen-tration (ppb)	Qual-ifier
1/16/2009	17	toluene	0	0	0.027	N/A	
1/17/2009	1	acetic acid	60	5.96	0.89	61	J
1/17/2009	1	α-pinene	60	5.96	0.08	2.4	J
1/17/2009	1	hexanal	60	5.96	0.038	1.5	J
1/17/2009	1	nonanal	60	5.96	0.078	2.3	J
1/17/2009	1	phenol	60	5.96	0.018	0.78	J
1/17/2009	1	tetradecane	60	5.96	0.036	0.74	J
1/17/2009	2	acetic acid	60	5.99	0.47	32	J
1/17/2009	2	α-pinene	60	5.99	0.056	1.7	J
1/17/2009	2	hexanal	60	5.99	0.028	1.1	J
1/17/2009	2	nonanal	60	5.99	0.059	1.7	J
1/17/2009	2	propanoic acid, 2-methyl	60	5.99	0.028	1.3	J
1/17/2009	2	tetradecane	60	5.99	0.027	0.56	J
1/17/2009	3	acetic acid	60	6.05	0.27	18	J
1/17/2009	3	α-pinene	60	6.05	0.064	1.9	J
1/17/2009	3	hexanal	60	6.05	0.037	1.5	J
1/17/2009	3	nonanal	60	6.05	0.072	2.1	J
1/17/2009	3	tetradecane	60	6.05	0.025	0.51	J
1/17/2009	4	acetic acid	60	6.04	0.49	33	J
1/17/2009	4	α-pinene	60	6.04	0.089	2.7	J
1/17/2009	4	hexanal	60	6.04	0.024	0.95	J
1/17/2009	4	tetradecane	60	6.04	0.028	0.57	J
1/17/2009	5	acetic acid	60	6.05	0.7	47	J
1/17/2009	5	α-pinene	60	6.05	0.11	3.3	J
1/17/2009	5	hexanal	60	6.05	0.036	1.4	J
1/17/2009	5	nonanal	60	6.05	0.066	1.9	J
1/17/2009	5	propanoic acid, 2-methyl	60	6.05	0.019	0.87	J
1/17/2009	5	tetradecane	60	6.05	0.029	0.59	J
1/17/2009	6	acetone	60	6.04	0.026	1.8	J
1/17/2009	6	α-pinene	60	6.04	0.054	1.6	J
1/17/2009	6	dichlorodifluormethane	60	6.04	0.028	0.94	J
1/17/2009	6	hexanal	60	6.04	0.029	1.2	J
1/17/2009	6	nonanal	60	6.04	0.048	1.4	J
1/17/2009	6	tetradecane	60	6.04	0.025	0.51	J
1/17/2009	7	acetic acid	60	6.05	0.42	28	J
1/17/2009	7	α-pinene	60	6.05	0.094	2.8	J
1/17/2009	7	dichlorodifluormethane	60	6.05	0.031	1.0	
1/17/2009	7	formic acid	60	6.05	0.022	1.9	J
1/17/2009	7	hexanal	60	6.05	0.026	1.0	J
1/17/2009	7	nonanal	60	6.05	0.052	1.5	J
1/17/2009	7	tetradecane	60	6.05	0.033	0.67	J
1/17/2009	8	acetic acid	60	6.01	0.55	37	J

Date	Trailer	Analyte	Sample Duration (minutes)	Sample Volume (liters)	Sample Mass (μg)	Concentration (ppb)	Qual-ifier
1/17/2009	8	α-pinene	60	6.01	0.08	2.4	J
1/17/2009	8	hexanal	60	6.01	0.038	1.5	J
1/17/2009	8	nonanal	60	6.01	0.084	2.4	J
1/17/2009	8	phenol	60	6.01	0.035	1.5	J
1/17/2009	8	tetradecane	60	6.01	0.062	1.3	J
1/17/2009	8	tridecane	60	6.01	0.018	0.40	J
1/17/2009	9	acetic acid	60	6.04	0.094	6.3	J
1/17/2009	9	acetone	60	6.04	0.067	4.7	
1/17/2009	9	α-pinene	60	6.04	0.12	3.6	J
1/17/2009	9	dichlorodifluormethane	60	6.04	0.036	1.2	
1/17/2009	9	hexanal	60	6.04	0.036	1.4	J
1/17/2009	9	methylene chloride	60	6.04	0.029	1.4	
1/17/2009	9	nonanal	60	6.04	0.071	2.0	J
1/17/2009	9	tetradecane	60	6.04	0.042	0.86	J
1/17/2009	10	acetic acid	60	6.04	0.83	56	J
1/17/2009	10	acetone	60	6.04	0.026	1.8	
1/17/2009	10	α-pinene	60	6.04	0.11	3.3	J
1/17/2009	10	hexanal	60	6.04	0.041	1.6	J
1/17/2009	10	nonanal	60	6.04	0.066	1.9	J
1/17/2009	10	propanoic acid, 2-methyl	60	6.04	0.021	0.96	J
1/17/2009	10	tetradecane	60	6.04	0.02	0.41	J
1/17/2009	11	α-pinene	60	6.07	0.11	3.3	J
1/17/2009	11	formic acid	60	6.07	0.057	5.0	J
1/17/2009	11	hexanal	60	6.07	0.037	1.5	J
1/17/2009	11	nonanal	60	6.07	0.068	1.9	J
1/17/2009	11	phenol	60	6.07	0.016	0.68	J
1/17/2009	11	tetradecane	60	6.07	0.031	0.63	J
1/17/2009	11	tridecane	60	6.07	0.016	0.35	J
1/17/2009	12	acetic acid	60	6.06	0.41	28	J
1/17/2009	12	α-pinene	60	6.06	0.071	2.1	J
1/17/2009	12	hexanal	60	6.06	0.031	1.2	J
1/17/2009	12	nonanal	60	6.06	0.057	1.6	J
1/17/2009	12	phenol	60	6.06	0.021	0.90	J
1/17/2009	12	propanoic acid, 2-methyl	60	6.06	0.021	0.96	J
1/17/2009	12	tetradecane	60	6.06	0.035	0.71	J
1/17/2009	13	acetic acid	60	6.03	0.34	23	J
1/17/2009	13	α-pinene	60	6.03	0.1	3.0	J
1/17/2009	13	hexanal	60	6.03	0.026	1.0	J
1/17/2009	13	nonanal	60	6.03	0.046	1.3	J
1/17/2009	13	tetradecane	60	6.03	0.025	0.51	J
1/17/2009	14	acetic acid	60	6.09	0.37	25	J
1/17/2009	14	α-pinene	60	6.09	0.082	2.4	J

Date	Trailer	Analyte	Sample Duration (minutes)	Sample Volume (liters)	Sample Mass (µg)	Concen-tration (ppb)	Qual-ifier
1/17/2009	14	hexanal	60	6.09	0.017	0.67	J
1/17/2009	14	nonanal	60	6.09	0.044	1.2	J
1/17/2009	14	tetradecane	60	6.09	0.037	0.75	J
1/17/2009	15	acetic acid	60	6.04	0.5	33.7	J
1/17/2009	15	α-pinene	60	6.04	0.11	3.3	J
1/17/2009	15	hexanal	60	6.04	0.045	1.8	J
1/17/2009	15	nonanal	60	6.04	0.055	1.6	J
1/17/2009	15	phenol	60	6.04	0.026	1.1	J
1/17/2009	15	propanoic acid, 2-methyl	60	6.04	0.02	0.92	J
1/17/2009	15	tetradecane	60	6.04	0.029	0.59	J
1/17/2009	16	acetaldehyde	60	6.04	0.016	1.5	J
1/17/2009	16	acetic acid	60	6.04	0.026	1.8	J
1/17/2009	16	acetonitrile	60	6.04	0.23	23	J
1/17/2009	16	butane, 2-methyl-	60	6.04	0.022	1.2	J
1/17/2009	16	nonanal	60	6.04	0.02	0.57	J
1/17/2009	17	acetic acid	0	0	0.017	N/A	
1/19/2009	4	acetic acid	60	6.03	0.53	36	J
1/19/2009	4	acetone	60	6.03	0.044	3.1	
1/19/2009	4	α-pinene	60	6.03	0.094	2.8	J
1/19/2009	4	hexanal	60	6.03	0.022	0.87	J
1/19/2009	4	nonanal	60	6.03	0.05	1.4	J
1/19/2009	4	tetradecane	60	6.03	0.04	0.82	J
1/19/2009	5	acetic acid	60	6.04	0.38	26	J
1/19/2009	5	α-pinene	60	6.04	0.084	2.5	J
1/19/2009	5	butane, 2-methyl-	60	6.04	0.069	3.9	J
1/19/2009	5	hexanal	60	6.04	0.024	0.95	J
1/19/2009	5	nonanal	60	6.04	0.05	1.4	J
1/19/2009	5	tetradecane	60	6.04	0.027	0.55	J
1/19/2009	6	acetic acid	60	6.04	0.26	18	J
1/19/2009	6	α-pinene	60	6.04	0.063	1.9	
1/19/2009	6	butane, 2-methyl-	60	6.04	0.069	3.9	J
1/19/2009	6	hexanal	60	6.04	0.017	0.67	J
1/19/2009	6	nonanal	60	6.04	0.06	1.7	J
1/19/2009	6	phenol	60	6.04	0.016	0.69	J
1/19/2009	6	tetradecane	60	6.04	0.041	0.84	J
1/19/2009	6	tridecane	60	6.04	0.017	0.37	J
1/19/2009	7	acetic acid	60	6.04	0.29	20	J
1/19/2009	7	acetone	60	6.04	0.03	2.1	
1/19/2009	7	α-pinene	60	6.04	0.073	2.2	J
1/19/2009	7	nonanal	60	6.04	0.039	1.1	
1/19/2009	7	phenol	60	6.04	0.017	0.73	J
1/19/2009	7	tetradecane	60	6.04	0.042	0.86	J

Date	Trailer	Analyte	Sample Duration (minutes)	Sample Volume (liters)	Sample Mass (μg)	Concen-tration (ppb)	Qual-ifier
1/19/2009	7	tridecane	60	6.04	0.019	0.42	J
1/19/2009	7	xylene	60	6.04	0.068	2.6	
1/19/2009	7	xylene	60	6.04	0.158	6.0	
1/19/2009	8	acetic acid	60	6.05	0.25	17	J
1/19/2009	8	acetone	60	6.05	0.11	7.7	
1/19/2009	8	α-pinene	60	6.05	0.073	2.2	J
1/19/2009	8	dichlorodifluormethane	60	6.05	0.05	1.7	
1/19/2009	8	ethanol	60	6.05	0.081	7.1	
1/19/2009	8	hexanal	60	6.05	0.022	0.87	J
1/19/2009	8	nonanal	60	6.05	0.044	1.3	J
1/19/2009	8	phenol	60	6.05	0.032	1.4	J
1/19/2009	8	tetradecane	60	6.05	0.049	1.0	J
1/19/2009	9	acetic acid	60	6.05	0.13	8.8	J
1/19/2009	9	acetone	60	6.05	0.035	2.4	
1/19/2009	9	nonanal	60	6.05	0.03	0.85	J
1/19/2009	10	acetone	60	6.05	1.2	84	
1/19/2009	10	α-pinene	60	6.05	0.055	1.6	J
1/19/2009	10	dichlorodifluormethane	60	6.05	0.046	1.5	
1/19/2009	10	ethanol	60	6.05	0.052	4.6	
1/19/2009	10	nonanal	60	6.05	0.039	1.1	J
1/19/2009	10	tetradecane	60	6.05	0.023	0.47	J
1/19/2009	11	acetic acid	60	6.05	1.1	74	J
1/19/2009	11	acetone	60	6.05	0.52	36	
1/19/2009	11	α-pinene	60	6.05	0.13	3.9	J
1/19/2009	11	dichlorodifluormethane	60	6.05	0.05	1.7	J
1/19/2009	11	formic acid	60	6.05	0.095	8.4	J
1/19/2009	11	hexanal	60	6.05	0.035	1.4	J
1/19/2009	11	isopropyl alcohol	60	6.05	0.027	1.8	J
1/19/2009	11	nonanal	60	6.05	0.085	2.4	J
1/19/2009	11	phenol	60	6.05	0.018	0.77	J
1/19/2009	11	propanoic acid, 2-methyl	60	6.05	0.049	2.3	J
1/19/2009	11	tetradecane	60	6.05	0.044	0.90	J
1/19/2009	12	acetaldehyde	60	6.05	0.3	28	J
1/19/2009	12	acetic acid	60	6.05	0.73	49	
1/19/2009	12	α-pinene	60	6.05	0.021	0.62	J
1/19/2009	12	dichlorodifluormethane	60	6.05	0.03	1.0	
1/19/2009	13	acetone	60	6.03	0.29	20	
1/19/2009	13	α-pinene	60	6.03	0.055	1.6	J
1/19/2009	13	dichlorodifluormethane	60	6.03	0.049	1.6	
1/19/2009	13	nonanal	60	6.03	0.026	0.74	J
1/19/2009	13	tetradecane	60	6.03	0.02	0.41	J
1/19/2009	14	acetone	60	6.03	0.14	9.8	

Date	Trailer	Analyte	Sample Duration (minutes)	Sample Volume (liters)	Sample Mass (µg)	Concen-tration (ppb)	Qual-ifier
1/19/2009	14	α-pinene	60	6.03	0.1	3.0	J
1/19/2009	14	dichlorodifluormethane	60	6.03	0.048	1.6	
1/19/2009	14	ethanol	60	6.03	0.059	5.2	
1/19/2009	14	hexanal	60	6.03	0.016	0.64	J
1/19/2009	14	nonanal	60	6.03	0.065	1.9	J
1/19/2009	14	tetradecane	60	6.03	0.045	0.92	J
1/19/2009	15	acetic acid	60	6.02	0.024	1.6	J
1/19/2009	15	acetone	60	6.02	0.14	9.8	
1/19/2009	15	α-pinene	60	6.02	0.082	2.4	J
1/19/2009	15	dichlorodifluormethane	60	6.02	0.044	1.5	
1/19/2009	15	ethanol	60	6.02	0.046	4.1	
1/19/2009	15	hexanal	60	6.02	0.02	0.79	J
1/19/2009	15	nonanal	60	6.02	0.076	2.2	J
1/19/2009	15	phenol	60	6.02	0.021	0.91	J
1/19/2009	15	tetradecane	60	6.02	0.042	0.86	J
1/19/2009	15	tridecane	60	6.02	0.017	0.37	J
1/19/2009	16	acetaldehyde	60	5.99	0.025	2.3	J
1/19/2009	16	acetic acid	60	5.99	0.028	1.9	J
1/19/2009	16	acetonitrile	60	5.99	0.032	3.2	J
1/19/2009	16	butane, 2-methyl-	60	5.99	0.056	3.2	J
1/19/2009	16	dichlorodifluormethane	60	5.99	0.03	1.0	
1/19/2009	16	nonanal	60	5.99	0.039	1.1	J
1/19/2009	17	acetaldehyde	0	0	0.022	N/A	J
1/28/2009	1	acetic acid	66	6.59	1.5	93	J
1/28/2009	1	acetone	66	6.59	0.03	1.9	
1/28/2009	1	α-pinene	66	6.59	0.15	4.1	J
1/28/2009	1	dichlorodifluormethane	66	6.59	0.029	0.89	
1/28/2009	1	hexanal	66	6.59	0.068	2.5	J
1/28/2009	1	methylene chloride	66	6.59	0.033	1.4	
1/28/2009	1	nonanal	66	6.59	0.11	2.9	J
1/28/2009	1	phenol	66	6.59	0.065	2.6	J
1/28/2009	1	tetradecane	66	6.59	0.071	1.3	J
1/28/2009	1	tridecane	66	6.59	0.047	0.95	J
1/28/2009	2	acetic acid	60	5.94	0.85	58	J
1/28/2009	2	α-pinene	60	5.94	0.14	4.2	J
1/28/2009	2	dibutyl phthalate	60	5.94	0.094	1.4	J
1/28/2009	2	ethanol	60	5.94	0.068	6.1	
1/28/2009	2	hexanal	60	5.94	0.044	1.8	J
1/28/2009	2	methylene chloride	60	5.94	0.038	1.8	
1/28/2009	2	nonanal	60	5.94	0.1	2.9	J
1/28/2009	2	phenol	60	5.94	0.036	1.6	J
1/28/2009	2	tetradecane	60	5.94	0.048	1.0	J

Date	Trailer	Analyte	Sample Duration (minutes)	Sample Volume (liters)	Sample Mass (μg)	Concen-tration (ppb)	Qual-ifier
1/28/2009	2	xylene	60	5.94	0.035	1.5	
1/28/2009	3	acetic acid	60	5.97	0.58	40	J
1/28/2009	3	acetone	60	5.97	0.095	6.7	
1/28/2009	3	α-pinene	60	5.97	0.13	3.9	J
1/28/2009	3	dibutyl phthalate	60	5.97	0.09	1.3	J
1/28/2009	3	dichlorodifluormethane	60	5.97	0.036	1.2	
1/28/2009	3	ethanol	60	5.97	0.032	2.9	
1/28/2009	3	methylene chloride	60	5.97	0.12	5.8	
1/28/2009	3	nonanal	60	5.97	0.06	1.7	J
1/28/2009	3	tetradecane	60	5.97	0.032	0.66	J
1/28/2009	4	acetic acid	60	5.97	0.34	23	J
1/28/2009	4	α-pinene	60	5.97	0.17	5.1	J
1/28/2009	4	dibutyl phthalate	60	5.97	0.48	7.1	J
1/28/2009	4	methylene chloride	60	5.97	0.051	2.5	
1/28/2009	4	nonanal	60	5.97	0.091	2.6	J
1/28/2009	5	acetic acid	60	5.96	0.86	59	J
1/28/2009	5	acetone	60	5.96	0.12	8.5	
1/28/2009	5	α-pinene	60	5.96	0.15	4.5	J
1/28/2009	5	dibutyl phthalate	60	5.96	0.3	4.4	J
1/28/2009	5	dichlorodifluormethane	60	5.96	0.032	1.1	
1/28/2009	5	hexanal	60	5.96	0.038	1.5	J
1/28/2009	5	methylene chloride	60	5.96	0.16	7.7	
1/28/2009	5	nonanal	60	5.96	0.08	2.3	J
1/28/2009	5	phenol	60	5.96	0.028	1.2	J
1/28/2009	5	tetradecane	60	5.96	0.045	0.93	J
1/28/2009	6	acetic acid	61	6.07	0.65	44	J
1/28/2009	6	acetone	61	6.07	0.17	12	
1/28/2009	6	α-pinene	61	6.07	0.1	3.0	
1/28/2009	6	dibutyl phthalate	61	6.07	0.16	2.3	J
1/28/2009	6	dichlorodifluormethane	61	6.07	0.025	0.83	
1/28/2009	6	hexanal	61	6.07	0.031	1.2	J
1/28/2009	6	methylene chloride	61	6.07	0.14	6.6	
1/28/2009	6	nonanal	61	6.07	0.082	2.3	J
1/28/2009	6	phenol	61	6.07	0.041	1.8	
1/28/2009	6	tetradecane	61	6.07	0.055	1.1	J
1/28/2009	6	tridecane	61	6.07	0.021	0.46	J
1/28/2009	7	acetic acid	64	6.38	0.24	15	J
1/28/2009	7	α-pinene	64	6.38	0.2	5.6	J
1/28/2009	7	dibutyl phthalate	64	6.38	0.16	2.2	J
1/28/2009	7	nonanal	64	6.38	0.052	1.4	J
1/28/2009	7	xylene	64	6.38	0.04	1.4	
1/28/2009	8	acetic acid	60	5.98	0.71	48	J

Date	Trailer	Analyte	Sample Duration (minutes)	Sample Volume (liters)	Sample Mass (µg)	Concentration (ppb)	Qual-ifier
1/28/2009	8	α-pinene	60	5.98	0.15	4.5	J
1/28/2009	8	dibutyl phthalate	60	5.98	0.19	2.8	J
1/28/2009	8	hexanal	60	5.98	0.043	1.7	J
1/28/2009	8	nonanal	60	5.98	0.056	1.6	J
1/28/2009	8	phenol	60	5.98	0.076	3.3	J
1/28/2009	8	tetradecane	60	5.98	0.099	2.0	J
1/28/2009	9	acetic acid	65	6.45	0.09	5.7	J
1/28/2009	9	α-pinene	65	6.45	0.026	0.72	J
1/28/2009	9	dibutyl phthalate	65	6.45	0.038	0.52	J
1/28/2009	9	nonanal	65	6.45	0.059	1.6	J
1/28/2009	10	acetic acid	65	6.46	0.51	32	J
1/28/2009	10	acetone	65	6.46	0.07	4.6	
1/28/2009	10	α-pinene	65	6.46	0.12	3.3	J
1/28/2009	10	dibutyl phthalate	65	6.46	0.065	0.88	J
1/28/2009	10	hexanal	65	6.46	0.025	0.93	J
1/28/2009	10	nonanal	65	6.46	0.052	1.4	J
1/28/2009	11	acetone	63	6.28	0.15	10	
1/28/2009	11	α-pinene	63	6.28	0.28	8.0	J
1/28/2009	11	dibutyl phthalate	63	6.28	0.092	1.3	J
1/28/2009	11	dichlorodifluormethane	63	6.28	0.037	1.2	
1/28/2009	11	formic acid	63	6.28	0.12	10	J
1/28/2009	11	hexanal	63	6.28	0.08	3.1	J
1/28/2009	11	isopropyl alcohol	63	6.28	0.25	16	
1/28/2009	11	methylene chloride	63	6.28	0.32	15	
1/28/2009	11	nonanal	63	6.28	0.17	4.7	J
1/28/2009	11	phenol	63	6.28	0.044	1.8	J
1/28/2009	11	tetradecane	63	6.28	0.07	1.4	J
1/28/2009	12	acetic acid	66	6.57	0.3	19	J
1/28/2009	12	acetone	66	6.57	0.21	13	
1/28/2009	12	α-pinene	66	6.57	0.045	1.2	J
1/28/2009	12	dibutyl phthalate	66	6.57	0.069	0.92	J
1/28/2009	12	isopropyl alcohol	66	6.57	0.13	8.1	J
1/28/2009	12	methylene chloride	66	6.57	0.11	4.8	
1/28/2009	12	nonanal	66	6.57	0.039	1.0	J
1/28/2009	12	tetradecane	66	6.57	0.027	0.51	J
1/28/2009	13	acetic acid	60	5.97	0.22	15	J
1/28/2009	13	acetone	60	5.97	0.58	41	
1/28/2009	13	α-pinene	60	5.97	0.19	5.7	J
1/28/2009	13	dibutyl phthalate	60	5.97	0.062	0.91	J
1/28/2009	13	isopropyl alcohol	60	5.97	0.092	6.3	
1/28/2009	13	methylene chloride	60	5.97	0.13	6.3	
1/28/2009	13	nonanal	60	5.97	0.043	1.2	J

Date	Trailer	Analyte	Sample Duration (minutes)	Sample Volume (liters)	Sample Mass (μg)	Concentration (ppb)	Qual-ifier
1/28/2009	13	tetradecane	60	5.97	0.035	0.72	J
1/28/2009	14	acetic acid	66	6.57	0.32	20	J
1/28/2009	14	acetone	66	6.57	0.042	2.7	
1/28/2009	14	α-pinene	66	6.57	0.15	4.1	J
1/28/2009	14	dibutyl phthalate	66	6.57	0.046	0.62	J
1/28/2009	14	hexanal	66	6.57	0.035	1.3	J
1/28/2009	14	isopropyl alcohol	66	6.57	0.056	3.5	
1/28/2009	14	methylene chloride	66	6.57	0.073	3.2	
1/28/2009	14	nonanal	66	6.57	0.051	1.3	J
1/28/2009	14	tetradecane	66	6.57	0.043	0.81	J
1/28/2009	15	acetic acid	60	5.98	0.72	49	J
1/28/2009	15	α-pinene	60	5.98	0.12	3.6	J
1/28/2009	15	hexanal	60	5.98	0.043	1.7	J
1/28/2009	15	nonanal	60	5.98	0.082	2.4	J
1/28/2009	15	phenol	60	5.98	0.03	1.3	J
1/28/2009	15	tetradecane	60	5.98	0.036	0.74	J
1/28/2009	16	acetic acid	63	6.28	0.027	1.8	J
1/28/2009	16	acetonitrile	63	6.28	0.097	9.2	J
1/28/2009	16	butane, 2-methyl-	63	6.28	0.024	1.3	J
1/28/2009	16	nonanal	63	6.28	0.02	0.55	J
3/5/2009	1	acetic acid	60	6.02	1.1	74	J
3/5/2009	1	acetone	60	6.02	0.041	2.9	
3/5/2009	1	α-pinene	60	6.02	0.24	7.2	J
3/5/2009	1	hexanal	60	6.02	0.082	3.3	J
3/5/2009	1	nonanal	60	6.02	0.18	5.1	J
3/5/2009	1	phenol	60	6.02	0.06	2.6	J
3/5/2009	1	tetradecane	60	6.02	0.11	2.3	J
3/5/2009	1	tridecane	60	6.02	0.034	0.75	J
3/5/2009	2	acetic acid	60	6.04	0.17	11	J
3/5/2009	2	acetone	60	6.04	0.14	9.8	
3/5/2009	2	α-pinene	60	6.04	0.2	6.0	J
3/5/2009	2	hexanal	60	6.04	0.068	2.7	J
3/5/2009	2	nonanal	60	6.04	0.24	6.8	J
3/5/2009	2	propanoic acid, 2-methyl	60	6.04	0.11	5.1	J
3/5/2009	2	tetradecane	60	6.04	0.061	1.3	J
3/5/2009	4	4-methyl-2-pentanone	60	6.02	0.028	1.1	J
3/5/2009	4	acetic acid	60	6.02	1.1	74	J
3/5/2009	4	acetone	60	6.02	0.05	3.5	
3/5/2009	4	α-pinene	60	6.02	0.28	8.4	J
3/5/2009	4	nonanal	60	6.02	0.086	2.5	J
3/5/2009	4	tetradecane	60	6.02	0.074	1.5	J
3/5/2009	5	acetic acid	60	6.05	0.1	6.7	J

Date	Trailer	Analyte	Sample Duration (minutes)	Sample Volume (liters)	Sample Mass (μg)	Concentration (ppb)	Qual-ifier
3/5/2009	5	acetone	60	6.05	0.094	6.6	
3/5/2009	5	α-pinene	60	6.05	0.27	8.0	J
3/5/2009	5	dichlorodifluormethane	60	6.05	0.045	1.5	
3/5/2009	5	hexanal	60	6.05	0.059	2.3	J
3/5/2009	5	nonanal	60	6.05	0.16	4.6	J
3/5/2009	5	tetradecane	60	6.05	0.056	1.1	J
3/5/2009	6	acetic acid	60	6.04	0.67	45	J
3/5/2009	6	acetone	60	6.04	0.045	3.1	
3/5/2009	6	α-pinene	60	6.04	0.17	5.1	J
3/5/2009	6	hexanal	60	6.04	0.048	1.9	J
3/5/2009	6	nonanal	60	6.04	0.21	6.0	J
3/5/2009	6	propanoic acid, 2-methyl	60	6.04	0.042	1.9	J
3/5/2009	6	tetradecane	60	6.04	0.11	2.3	J
3/5/2009	7	acetic acid	60	6.04	0.29	20	J
3/5/2009	7	acetone	60	6.04	0.056	3.9	
3/5/2009	7	α-pinene	60	6.04	0.27	8.0	J
3/5/2009	7	hexanal	60	6.04	0.048	1.9	J
3/5/2009	7	nonanal	60	6.04	0.13	3.7	J
3/5/2009	7	tetradecane	60	6.04	0.08	1.6	J
3/5/2009	8	α-pinene	60	6.05	0.23	6.8	J
3/5/2009	8	hexanal	60	6.05	0.07	2.8	J
3/5/2009	8	nonanal	60	6.05	0.18	5.1	J
3/5/2009	8	tetradecane	60	6.05	0.16	3.3	J
3/5/2009	9	acetic acid	60	6.04	0.065	4.4	J
3/5/2009	9	acetone	60	6.04	0.036	2.5	
3/5/2009	9	α-pinene	60	6.04	0.02	0.59	J
3/5/2009	9	hexanal	60	6.04	0.025	0.99	J
3/5/2009	9	nonanal	60	6.04	0.088	2.5	J
3/5/2009	10	acetic acid	60	6.03	0.42	28	J
3/5/2009	10	acetone	60	6.03	0.24	16.8	
3/5/2009	10	α-pinene	60	6.03	0.17	5.1	J
3/5/2009	10	dichlorodifluormethane	60	6.03	0.048	1.6	
3/5/2009	10	nonanal	60	6.03	0.089	2.5	J
3/5/2009	10	tetradecane	60	6.03	0.025	0.51	J
3/5/2009	11	acetic acid	60	6.03	1.4	95	J
3/5/2009	11	acetone	60	6.03	0.12	8.4	
3/5/2009	11	α-pinene	60	6.03	0.3	8.9	J
3/5/2009	11	formic acid	60	6.03	0.071	6.3	J
3/5/2009	11	hexanal	60	6.03	0.078	3.1	J
3/5/2009	11	nonanal	60	6.03	0.16	4.6	J
3/5/2009	11	propanoic acid, 2-methyl	60	6.03	0.12	5.5	J
3/5/2009	11	styrene	60	6.03	0.067	2.6	

Date	Trailer	Analyte	Sample Duration (minutes)	Sample Volume (liters)	Sample Mass (µg)	Concen-tration (ppb)	Qual -ifier
3/5/2009	11	tetradecane	60	6.03	0.054	1.1	J
3/5/2009	12	acetic acid	60	6.02	0.23	16	J
3/5/2009	12	acetone	60	6.02	0.25	17	
3/5/2009	12	α-pinene	60	6.02	0.055	1.6	J
3/5/2009	12	nonanal	60	6.02	0.049	1.4	J
3/5/2009	12	tetradecane	60	6.02	0.018	0.37	J
3/5/2009	13	acetone	60	6.03	0.18	13	
3/5/2009	13	α-pinene	60	6.03	0.16	4.8	J
3/5/2009	13	dichlorodifluormethane	60	6.03	0.037	1.2	
3/5/2009	13	hexanal	60	6.03	0.02	0.79	J
3/5/2009	13	nonanal	60	6.03	0.057	1.6	J
3/5/2009	13	tetradecane	60	6.03	0.027	0.55	J
3/5/2009	14	acetic acid	60	6.03	0.61	41	J
3/5/2009	14	acetone	60	6.03	0.057	4.0	
3/5/2009	14	α-pinene	60	6.03	0.24	7.1	J
3/5/2009	14	dichlorodifluormethane	60	6.03	0.032	1.1	
3/5/2009	14	hexanal	60	6.03	0.032	1.3	J
3/5/2009	14	tetradecane	60	6.03	0.097	2.0	J
3/5/2009	15	acetic acid	60	6.03	0.7	47	J
3/5/2009	15	acetone	60	6.03	0.056	3.9	
3/5/2009	15	α-pinene	60	6.03	0.16	4.8	J
3/5/2009	15	hexanal	60	6.03	0.047	1.9	J
3/5/2009	15	nonanal	60	6.03	0.14	4.0	J
3/5/2009	15	tetradecane	60	6.03	0.052	1.1	J
3/5/2009	16	acetic acid	60	6.04	0.024	1.6	J
3/5/2009	16	acetone	60	6.04	0.034	2.4	
3/5/2009	16	nonanal	60	6.04	0.054	1.5	J
3/5/2009	17	acetone	0	0	0.026	N/A	
3/19/2009	1	α-pinene	60	6.08	0.41	12	J
3/19/2009	1	hexanal	60	6.08	0.17	6.7	J
3/19/2009	1	nonanal	60	6.08	0.33	9.3	J
3/19/2009	1	tetradecane	60	6.08	0.18	3.7	J
3/19/2009	2	acetic acid	60	6.08	1.2	80	J
3/19/2009	2	acetone	60	6.08	0.19	13	
3/19/2009	2	α-pinene	60	6.08	0.4	12	J
3/19/2009	2	dibutyl phthalate	60	6.08	0.27	3.9	J
3/19/2009	2	dichlorodifluormethane	60	6.08	0.025	0.83	
3/19/2009	2	hexanal	60	6.08	0.13	5.1	J
3/19/2009	2	nonanal	60	6.08	0.35	9.9	
3/19/2009	2	styrene	60	6.08	0.039	1.5	
3/19/2009	2	tetradecane	60	6.08	0.19	3.9	J
3/19/2009	4	acetic acid	60	6.09	0.97	65	J

Date	Trailer	Analyte	Sample Duration (minutes)	Sample Volume (liters)	Sample Mass (μg)	Concentration (ppb)	Qual-ifier
3/19/2009	4	acetone	60	6.09	0.12	8.3	
3/19/2009	4	α-pinene	60	6.09	0.42	12.4	J
3/19/2009	4	dibutyl phthalate	60	6.09	1.5	22	J
3/19/2009	4	nonanal	60	6.09	0.26	7.3	J
3/19/2009	5	acetic acid	60	6.10	0.9	60	J
3/19/2009	5	acetone	60	6.10	0.077	5.3	
3/19/2009	5	α-pinene	60	6.10	0.35	10.3	J
3/19/2009	5	dibutyl phthalate	60	6.10	1.1	15.8	J
3/19/2009	5	dichlorodifluormethane	60	6.10	0.033	1.1	
3/19/2009	5	hexanal	60	6.10	0.093	3.7	J
3/19/2009	5	nonanal	60	6.10	0.2	5.6	J
3/19/2009	6	acetic acid	60	6.10	0.84	56	J
3/19/2009	6	acetone	60	6.10	0.095	6.6	
3/19/2009	6	α-pinene	60	6.10	0.24	7.1	J
3/19/2009	6	dibutyl phthalate	60	6.10	0.76	11	J
3/19/2009	6	dichlorodifluormethane	60	6.10	0.029	0.96	
3/19/2009	6	hexanal	60	6.10	0.11	4.3	J
3/19/2009	6	nonanal	60	6.10	0.17	4.8	J
3/19/2009	6	tetradecane	60	6.10	0.069	1.4	J
3/19/2009	7	acetic acid	60	6.12	0.56	37	J
3/19/2009	7	acetone	60	6.12	0.046	3.2	
3/19/2009	7	α-pinene	60	6.12	0.41	12	J
3/19/2009	7	dibutyl phthalate	60	6.12	0.47	6.8	J
3/19/2009	7	tetradecane	60	6.12	0.099	2.0	J
3/19/2009	8	acetic acid	60	6.08	1.9	130	J
3/19/2009	8	acetone	60	6.08	0.13	9.0	
3/19/2009	8	α-pinene	60	6.08	0.32	9.5	J
3/19/2009	8	dibutyl phthalate	60	6.08	0.31	4.5	J
3/19/2009	8	dichlorodifluormethane	60	6.08	0.041	1.4	
3/19/2009	8	ethanol	60	6.08	0.066	5.8	
3/19/2009	8	hexanal	60	6.08	0.12	4.7	J
3/19/2009	8	nonanal	60	6.08	0.18	5.1	J
3/19/2009	8	phenol	60	6.08	0.13	5.6	J
3/19/2009	8	styrene	60	6.08	0.025	0.97	
3/19/2009	8	tetradecane	60	6.08	0.15	3.0	J
3/19/2009	9	acetic acid	60	6.11	0.11	7.3	J
3/19/2009	9	acetone	60	6.11	0.063	4.3	
3/19/2009	9	α-pinene	60	6.11	0.048	1.4	J
3/19/2009	9	dibutyl phthalate	60	6.11	0.65	9.4	J
3/19/2009	9	dichlorodifluormethane	60	6.11	0.028	0.93	
3/19/2009	9	nonanal	60	6.11	0.081	2.3	J
3/19/2009	10	acetic acid	60	6.10	0.59	39	J

Date	Trailer	Analyte	Sample Duration (minutes)	Sample Volume (liters)	Sample Mass (µg)	Concentration (ppb)	Qual-ifier
3/19/2009	10	acetone	60	6.10	0.16	11	
3/19/2009	10	α-pinene	60	6.10	0.24	7.1	J
3/19/2009	10	dibutyl phthalate	60	6.10	0.57	8.2	J
3/19/2009	10	dichlorodifluormethane	60	6.10	0.033	1.1	
3/19/2009	10	nonanal	60	6.10	0.1	2.8	J
3/19/2009	11	acetic acid	60	6.10	1.2	80	J
3/19/2009	11	acetone	60	6.10	0.33	23	
3/19/2009	11	α-pinene	60	6.10	0.48	14	J
3/19/2009	11	dibutyl phthalate	60	6.10	0.59	8.5	J
3/19/2009	11	formic acid	60	6.10	0.1	8.7	J
3/19/2009	11	hexanal	60	6.10	0.11	4.3	J
3/19/2009	11	isopropyl alcohol	60	6.10	0.026	1.7	
3/19/2009	11	nonanal	60	6.10	0.21	5.9	J
3/19/2009	11	propanoic acid, 2-methyl	60	6.10	0.27	12	J
3/19/2009	11	styrene	60	6.10	0.05	1.9	
3/19/2009	12	acetic acid	60	6.10	0.45	30	J
3/19/2009	12	acetone	60	6.10	1	69	
3/19/2009	12	α-pinene	60	6.10	0.1	2.9	J
3/19/2009	12	dibutyl phthalate	60	6.10	0.54	7.8	J
3/19/2009	12	dichlorodifluormethane	60	6.10	0.047	1.6	
3/19/2009	12	nonanal	60	6.10	0.057	1.6	J
3/19/2009	12	tetradecane	60	6.10	0.032	0.65	J
3/19/2009	13	acetic acid	60	6.11	0.31	21	J
3/19/2009	13	acetone	60	6.11	0.11	7.6	
3/19/2009	13	α-pinene	60	6.11	0.25	7.4	J
3/19/2009	13	dibutyl phthalate	60	6.11	0.47	6.8	J
3/19/2009	13	nonanal	60	6.11	0.067	1.9	J
3/19/2009	14	acetic acid	60	6.15	0.7	46	J
3/19/2009	14	acetone	60	6.15	0.043	2.9	
3/19/2009	14	α-pinene	60	6.15	0.37	11	J
3/19/2009	14	dibutyl phthalate	60	6.15	0.27	3.9	J
3/19/2009	14	dichlorodifluormethane	60	6.15	0.03	0.99	
3/19/2009	14	hexanal	60	6.15	0.087	3.4	J
3/19/2009	14	nonanal	60	6.15	0.12	3.4	J
3/19/2009	14	tetradecane	60	6.15	0.081	1.6	J
3/19/2009	15	acetone	60	6.11	0.038	2.6	
3/19/2009	15	α-pinene	60	6.11	0.25	7.3	J
3/19/2009	15	dibutyl phthalate	60	6.11	0.43	6.2	J
3/19/2009	15	formic acid	60	6.11	0.15	13	J
3/19/2009	15	hexanal	60	6.11	0.077	3.0	J
3/19/2009	15	nonanal	60	6.11	0.15	4.2	J
3/19/2009	15	tetradecane	60	6.11	0.065	1.3	J

Date	Trailer	Analyte	Sample Duration (minutes)	Sample Volume (liters)	Sample Mass (μg)	Concen-tration (ppb)	Qual-ifier
3/19/2009	16	acetic acid	60	6.11	0.017	1.1	J
3/19/2009	16	dibutyl phthalate	60	6.11	0.15	2.2	J
3/19/2009	16	hexanal	60	6.11	0.018	0.71	J
3/19/2009	16	nonanal	60	6.11	0.066	1.9	J
3/19/2009	17	butane, 2-methyl-	0	0	0.028	N/A	J
3/19/2009	17	dibutyl phthalate	0	0	0.19	N/A	J
4/2/2009	1	4-methyl-2-pentanone	105	10.5	0.043	1.0	
4/2/2009	1	acetic acid	105	10.5	1.4	54	J
4/2/2009	1	α-pinene	105	10.5	0.34	5.8	J
4/2/2009	1	formic acid	105	10.5	0.17	8.6	J
4/2/2009	1	hexanal	105	10.5	0.14	3.2	J
4/2/2009	1	methylene chloride	105	10.5	0.047	1.3	
4/2/2009	1	nonanal	105	10.5	0.28	4.6	J
4/2/2009	1	propanoic acid, 2-methyl	105	10.5	0.2	5.3	J
4/2/2009	1	tetradecane	105	10.5	0.12	1.4	J
4/2/2009	2	acetic acid	105	10.6	1.6	61	J
4/2/2009	2	α-pinene	105	10.6	0.42	7.1	J
4/2/2009	2	hexanal	105	10.6	0.13	2.9	J
4/2/2009	2	methylene chloride	105	10.6	0.032	0.87	
4/2/2009	2	nonanal	105	10.6	0.27	4.4	J
4/2/2009	2	propanoic acid, 2-methyl	105	10.6	0.19	5.0	J
4/2/2009	2	styrene	105	10.6	0.05	1.1	
4/2/2009	4	acetic acid	105	10.5	0.1	3.9	J
4/2/2009	4	α-pinene	105	10.5	0.1	1.7	J
4/2/2009	4	styrene	105	10.5	0.027	0.60	
4/2/2009	5	acetic acid	105	10.5	0.29	11	J
4/2/2009	5	α-pinene	105	10.5	0.38	6.5	J
4/2/2009	5	hexanal	105	10.5	0.091	2.1	J
4/2/2009	5	nonanal	105	10.5	0.17	2.8	J
4/2/2009	5	propanoic acid, 2-methyl	105	10.5	0.074	2.0	J
4/2/2009	5	tetradecane	105	10.5	0.041	0.48	J
4/2/2009	6	acetic acid	105	10.6	0.93	36	J
4/2/2009	6	α-pinene	105	10.6	0.25	4.3	J
4/2/2009	6	hexanal	105	10.6	0.099	2.3	J
4/2/2009	6	nonanal	105	10.6	0.15	2.4	J
4/2/2009	6	phenol	105	10.6	0.078	1.9	J
4/2/2009	6	propanoic acid, 2-methyl	105	10.6	0.069	1.8	J
4/2/2009	6	tetradecane	105	10.6	0.084	0.98	J
4/2/2009	7	acetic acid	105	10.5	0.92	36	J
4/2/2009	7	α-pinene	105	10.5	0.43	7.4	J
4/2/2009	7	hexanal	105	10.5	0.067	1.5	J
4/2/2009	7	phenol	105	10.5	0.1	2.5	J

Date	Trailer	Analyte	Sample Duration (minutes)	Sample Volume (liters)	Sample Mass (μg)	Concen-tration (ppb)	Qual-ifier
4/2/2009	7	propanoic acid, 2-methyl	105	10.5	0.2	5.3	J
4/2/2009	7	styrene	105	10.5	0.035	0.78	
4/2/2009	7	tetradecane	105	10.5	0.12	1.4	J
4/2/2009	8	4-methyl-2-pentanone	105	10.5	0.025	0.58	
4/2/2009	8	acetic acid	105	10.5	1.6	62	J
4/2/2009	8	α-pinene	105	10.5	0.43	7.3	J
4/2/2009	8	hexanal	105	10.5	0.099	2.3	J
4/2/2009	8	propanoic acid, 2-methyl	105	10.5	0.25	6.6	J
4/2/2009	8	styrene	105	10.5	0.046	1.0	
4/2/2009	8	tetradecane	105	10.5	0.13	1.5	J
4/2/2009	9	acetic acid	105	10.5	0.21	8.1	J
4/2/2009	9	acetone	105	10.5	0.08	3.2	
4/2/2009	9	α-pinene	105	10.5	0.077	1.3	J
4/2/2009	9	formic acid	105	10.5	0.018	0.91	J
4/2/2009	9	hexanal	105	10.5	0.036	0.82	J
4/2/2009	9	nonanal	105	10.5	0.095	1.6	J
4/2/2009	9	styrene	105	10.5	0.03	0.67	
4/2/2009	9	tetradecane	105	10.5	0.017	0.20	J
4/2/2009	10	acetic acid	107	10.7	0.82	31.2	J
4/2/2009	10	acetone	107	10.7	0.72	28	
4/2/2009	10	α-pinene	107	10.7	0.31	5.2	J
4/2/2009	10	hexanal	107	10.7	0.06	1.3	J
4/2/2009	10	methylene chloride	107	10.7	0.033	0.89	
4/2/2009	10	nonanal	107	10.7	0.098	1.6	J
4/2/2009	10	pentanal	107	10.7	0.028	0.74	J
4/2/2009	10	propanoic acid, 2-methyl	107	10.7	0.029	0.75	J
4/2/2009	10	styrene	107	10.7	0.043	0.94	
4/2/2009	10	tetradecane	107	10.7	0.03	0.35	J
4/2/2009	10	toluene	107	10.7	0.027	0.67	
4/2/2009	11	4-methyl-2-pentanone	105	10.6	0.048	1.1	
4/2/2009	11	acetone	105	10.6	0.23	9.2	
4/2/2009	11	α-pinene	105	10.6	0.46	7.8	J
4/2/2009	11	ethanol	105	10.6	0.033	1.7	
4/2/2009	11	hexanal	105	10.6	0.11	2.5	J
4/2/2009	11	isopropyl alcohol	105	10.6	0.026	1.0	
4/2/2009	11	methylene chloride	105	10.6	0.037	1.0	
4/2/2009	11	nonanal	105	10.6	0.25	4.1	J
4/2/2009	11	propanoic acid, 2-methyl	105	10.6	0.12	3.2	J
4/2/2009	11	styrene	105	10.6	0.068	1.5	
4/2/2009	11	tetradecane	105	10.6	0.099	1.2	J
4/2/2009	12	acetic acid	105	10.6	0.65	25	J
4/2/2009	12	α-pinene	105	10.6	0.16	2.7	J

Date	Trailer	Analyte	Sample Duration (minutes)	Sample Volume (liters)	Sample Mass (μg)	Concen-tration (ppb)	Qual-ifier
4/2/2009	12	hexanal	105	10.6	0.036	0.82	
4/2/2009	12	nonanal	105	10.6	0.077	1.3	J
4/2/2009	12	phenol	105	10.6	0.031	0.76	J
4/2/2009	12	propanoic acid, 2-methyl	105	10.6	0.042	1.1	J
4/2/2009	12	tetradecane	105	10.6	0.036	0.42	J
4/2/2009	13	acetone	105	10.6	1.2	48	
4/2/2009	13	α-pinene	105	10.6	0.33	5.6	J
4/2/2009	13	dichlorodifluormethane	105	10.6	0.031	0.59	
4/2/2009	13	ethanol	105	10.6	0.071	3.6	
4/2/2009	13	hexanal	105	10.6	0.037	0.84	J
4/2/2009	13	isopropyl alcohol	105	10.6	0.026	1.0	
4/2/2009	13	methylene chloride	105	10.6	0.055	1.5	
4/2/2009	13	nonanal	105	10.6	0.071	1.2	J
4/2/2009	13	propanoic acid, 2-methyl	105	10.6	0.033	0.87	J
4/2/2009	13	tetradecane	105	10.6	0.039	0.46	J
4/2/2009	14	acetic acid	122	12.3	0.83	28	J
4/2/2009	14	α-pinene	122	12.3	0.54	7.9	J
4/2/2009	14	methylene chloride	122	12.3	0.074	1.7	
4/2/2009	14	nonanal	122	12.3	0.16	2.2	J
4/2/2009	14	propanoic acid, 2-methyl	122	12.3	0.19	4.3	J
4/2/2009	14	tetradecane	122	12.3	0.082	0.82	J
4/2/2009	15	acetic acid	105	10.5	1.7	66	J
4/2/2009	15	α-pinene	105	10.5	0.27	4.6	J
4/2/2009	15	formic acid	105	10.5	0.085	4.3	J
4/2/2009	15	hexanal	105	10.5	0.077	1.8	J
4/2/2009	15	nonanal	105	10.5	0.18	2.9	J
4/2/2009	15	propanoic acid, 2-methyl	105	10.5	0.086	2.3	J
4/2/2009	16	acetic acid	106	10.7	0.082	3.1	J
4/2/2009	16	methylene chloride	106	10.7	0.074	2.0	
4/2/2009	17	methylene chloride	0	0	0.042	N/A	J
4/16/2009	1	α-pinene	60	6.05	0.16	4.8	J
4/16/2009	1	nonanal	60	6.05	0.16	4.6	J
4/16/2009	1	tetradecane	60	6.05	0.053	1.1	J
4/16/2009	2	acetone	60	6.04	0.041	2.9	
4/16/2009	2	α-pinene	60	6.04	0.19	5.7	J
4/16/2009	2	formic acid	60	6.04	0.13	11	J
4/16/2009	2	hexanal	60	6.04	0.079	3.1	J
4/16/2009	2	nonanal	60	6.04	0.18	5.1	J
4/16/2009	2	phenol	60	6.04	0.034	1.5	J
4/16/2009	2	tetradecane	60	6.04	0.062	1.3	J
4/16/2009	4	acetic acid	60	6.07	0.76	51	J
4/16/2009	4	α-pinene	60	6.07	0.26	7.7	J

164

Date	Trailer	Analyte	Sample Duration (minutes)	Sample Volume (liters)	Sample Mass (µg)	Concentration (ppb)	Qual-ifier
4/16/2009	4	hexanal	60	6.07	0.062	2.4	J
4/16/2009	4	nonanal	60	6.07	0.14	4.0	J
4/16/2009	4	propanoic acid, 2-methyl	60	6.07	0.033	1.5	J
4/16/2009	4	tetradecane	60	6.07	0.054	1.1	J
4/16/2009	5	acetic acid	60	6.09	1	67	J
4/16/2009	5	α-pinene	60	6.09	0.22	6.5	J
4/16/2009	5	formic acid	60	6.09	0.16	14	J
4/16/2009	5	hexanal	60	6.09	0.061	2.4	J
4/16/2009	5	nonanal	60	6.09	0.14	4.0	J
4/16/2009	5	tetradecane	60	6.09	0.041	0.83	J
4/16/2009	6	acetic acid	60	6.08	0.7	47	J
4/16/2009	6	acetone	60	6.08	0.039	2.7	
4/16/2009	6	α-pinene	60	6.08	0.14	4.1	J
4/16/2009	6	hexanal	60	6.08	0.056	2.2	J
4/16/2009	6	nonanal	60	6.08	0.13	3.7	J
4/16/2009	6	propanoic acid, 2-methyl	60	6.08	0.034	1.5	J
4/16/2009	6	tetradecane	60	6.08	0.05	1.0	J
4/16/2009	7	acetic acid	60	6.08	0.86	58	J
4/16/2009	7	α-pinene	60	6.08	0.21	6.2	J
4/16/2009	7	hexanal	60	6.08	0.025	0.98	J
4/16/2009	7	phenol	60	6.08	0.037	1.6	J
4/16/2009	7	propanoic acid, 2-methyl	60	6.08	0.026	1.2	J
4/16/2009	7	tetradecane	60	6.08	0.059	1.2	J
4/16/2009	8	acetic acid	60	6.12	0.99	66	J
4/16/2009	8	acetone	60	6.12	0.35	24	
4/16/2009	8	α-pinene	60	6.12	0.19	5.6	J
4/16/2009	8	dichlorodifluormethane	60	6.12	0.05	1.7	
4/16/2009	8	ethanol	60	6.12	0.27	23	
4/16/2009	8	hexanal	60	6.12	0.18	7.0	
4/16/2009	8	isopropyl alcohol	60	6.12	0.1	6.7	
4/16/2009	8	nonanal	60	6.12	0.26	7.3	J
4/16/2009	8	toluene	60	6.12	0.026	1.1	
4/16/2009	9	acetic acid	60	6.06	0.15	10	J
4/16/2009	9	acetone	60	6.06	0.071	4.9	
4/16/2009	9	α-pinene	60	6.06	0.03	0.89	J
4/16/2009	9	ethanol	60	6.06	0.1	8.8	
4/16/2009	9	hexanal	60	6.06	0.032	1.3	J
4/16/2009	9	nonanal	60	6.06	0.071	2.0	J
4/16/2009	10	acetic acid	60	6.08	0.45	30	J
4/16/2009	10	α-pinene	60	6.08	0.14	4.1	J
4/16/2009	10	formic acid	60	6.08	0.033	2.9	J
4/16/2009	10	hexanal	60	6.08	0.022	0.87	J

Date	Trailer	Analyte	Sample Duration (minutes)	Sample Volume (liters)	Sample Mass (µg)	Concentration (ppb)	Qual-ifier
4/16/2009	10	nonanal	60	6.08	0.079	2.2	J
4/16/2009	10	tetradecane	60	6.08	0.02	0.41	J
4/16/2009	11	acetic acid	60	6.08	1.5	100	J
4/16/2009	11	α-pinene	60	6.08	0.26	7.7	J
4/16/2009	11	formic acid	60	6.08	0.056	4.9	J
4/16/2009	11	hexanal	60	6.08	0.063	2.5	J
4/16/2009	11	nonanal	60	6.08	0.15	4.2	J
4/16/2009	11	propanoic acid, 2-methyl	60	6.08	0.18	8.2	J
4/16/2009	11	styrene	60	6.08	0.031	1.2	
4/16/2009	11	tetradecane	60	6.08	0.041	0.83	J
4/16/2009	12	acetic acid	60	6.07	0.34	23	J
4/16/2009	12	acetone	60	6.07	0.73	51	
4/16/2009	12	α-pinene	60	6.07	0.058	1.7	J
4/16/2009	12	dichlorodifluormethane	60	6.07	0.043	1.4	
4/16/2009	12	ethanol	60	6.07	0.031	2.7	
4/16/2009	12	formic acid	60	6.07	0.017	1.5	J
4/16/2009	12	hexanal	60	6.07	0.02	0.79	J
4/16/2009	12	nonanal	60	6.07	0.05	1.4	J
4/16/2009	12	tetradecane	60	6.07	0.016	0.32	J
4/16/2009	13	4-methyl-2-pentanone	60	6.08	0.042	1.7	J
4/16/2009	13	acetic acid	60	6.08	0.071	4.8	J
4/16/2009	13	acetone	60	6.08	0.2	14	
4/16/2009	13	α-pinene	60	6.08	0.18	5.3	J
4/16/2009	13	nonanal	60	6.08	0.037	1.1	J
4/16/2009	14	acetic acid	60	6.09	0.34	23	J
4/16/2009	14	acetone	60	6.09	0.058	4.0	
4/16/2009	14	α-pinene	60	6.09	0.19	5.6	J
4/16/2009	14	hexanal	60	6.09	0.043	1.7	J
4/16/2009	14	nonanal	60	6.09	0.085	2.4	J
4/16/2009	14	propanoic acid, 2-methyl	60	6.09	0.034	1.6	J
4/16/2009	14	tetradecane	60	6.09	0.035	0.71	J
4/16/2009	15	acetic acid	60	6.07	0.77	52	J
4/16/2009	15	α-pinene	60	6.07	0.14	4.1	J
4/16/2009	15	formic acid	60	6.07	0.043	3.8	J
4/16/2009	15	hexanal	60	6.07	0.045	1.8	J
4/16/2009	15	nonanal	60	6.07	0.15	4.2	J
4/16/2009	15	tetradecane	60	6.07	0.044	0.89	J
4/16/2009	16	acetone	60	6.10	0.056	3.9	
4/16/2009	16	ethanol	60	6.10	0.035	3.1	
4/16/2009	16	nonanal	60	6.10	0.067	1.9	J
5/6/2009	1	acetic acid	60	6.11	0.51	34	J
5/6/2009	1	α-pinene	60	6.11	0.29	8.5	J

Date	Trailer	Analyte	Sample Duration (minutes)	Sample Volume (liters)	Sample Mass (μg)	Concen-tration (ppb)	Qual-ifier
5/6/2009	1	hexanal	60	6.11	0.082	3.2	J
5/6/2009	1	nonanal	60	6.11	0.13	3.7	J
5/6/2009	1	tridecane	60	6.11	0.028	0.61	
5/6/2009	2	acetic acid	60	6.11	1.2	80	J
5/6/2009	2	α-pinene	60	6.11	0.26	7.6	J
5/6/2009	2	hexanal	60	6.11	0.06	2.4	J
5/6/2009	2	nonanal	60	6.11	0.13	3.7	J
5/6/2009	2	propanoic acid, 2-methyl	60	6.11	0.085	3.9	J
5/6/2009	2	styrene	60	6.11	0.049	1.9	
5/6/2009	2	tetradecane	60	6.11	0.071	1.4	J
5/6/2009	3	acetic acid	60	6.08	0.4	27	J
5/6/2009	3	acetone	60	6.08	0.029	2.0	
5/6/2009	3	α-pinene	60	6.08	0.2	5.9	J
5/6/2009	3	nonanal	60	6.08	0.088	2.5	J
5/6/2009	3	tetradecane	60	6.08	0.057	1.2	J
5/6/2009	4	acetic acid	60	6.08	0.75	50	J
5/6/2009	4	acetone	60	6.08	0.043	3.0	
5/6/2009	4	α-pinene	60	6.08	0.36	11	J
5/6/2009	4	nonanal	60	6.08	0.089	2.5	J
5/6/2009	4	phenol	60	6.08	0.036	1.5	J
5/6/2009	4	tetradecane	60	6.08	0.07	1.4	J
5/6/2009	4	tridecane	60	6.08	0.026	0.57	J
5/6/2009	5	acetic acid	60	6.06	1	67	J
5/6/2009	5	acetone	60	6.06	0.04	2.8	
5/6/2009	5	α-pinene	60	6.06	0.43	13	J
5/6/2009	5	dichlorodifluormethane	60	6.06	0.084	2.8	
5/6/2009	5	formic acid	60	6.06	0.065	5.7	J
5/6/2009	5	nonanal	60	6.06	0.12	3.4	J
5/6/2009	5	phenol	60	6.06	0.044	1.9	J
5/6/2009	5	styrene	60	6.06	0.03	1.2	
5/6/2009	5	tetradecane	60	6.06	0.079	1.6	J
5/6/2009	6	acetic acid	60	6.06	0.3	20	J
5/6/2009	6	acetone	60	6.06	0.46	32	
5/6/2009	6	α-pinene	60	6.06	0.25	7.4	J
5/6/2009	6	dichlorodifluormethane	60	6.06	0.12	4.0	
5/6/2009	6	nonanal	60	6.06	0.13	3.7	J
5/6/2009	6	propanoic acid, 2-methyl	60	6.06	0.041	1.9	J
5/6/2009	6	tetradecane	60	6.06	0.081	1.7	J
5/6/2009	7	acetic acid	60	6.03	0.45	30	J
5/6/2009	7	acetone	60	6.03	0.044	3.1	
5/6/2009	7	α-pinene	60	6.03	0.3	8.9	J
5/6/2009	7	dichlorodifluormethane	60	6.03	0.081	2.7	

Date	Trailer	Analyte	Sample Duration (minutes)	Sample Volume (liters)	Sample Mass (μg)	Concen-tration (ppb)	Qual-ifier
5/6/2009	7	nonanal	60	6.03	0.1	2.9	J
5/6/2009	7	phenol	60	6.03	0.038	1.6	J
5/6/2009	7	propanoic acid, 2-methyl	60	6.03	0.04	1.8	J
5/6/2009	7	styrene	60	6.03	0.034	1.3	
5/6/2009	7	tetradecane	60	6.03	0.072	1.5	J
5/6/2009	8	acetic acid	60	6.06	0.15	10	J
5/6/2009	8	acetone	60	6.06	0.057	4.0	
5/6/2009	8	α-pinene	60	6.06	0.24	7.1	J
5/6/2009	8	nonanal	60	6.06	0.14	34.0	J
5/6/2009	8	phenol	60	6.06	0.042	1.8	J
5/6/2009	8	propanoic acid, 2-methyl	60	6.06	0.13	56.0	J
5/6/2009	8	styrene	60	6.06	0.027	1.1	
5/6/2009	8	tetradecane	60	6.06	0.075	1.5	J
5/6/2009	9	4-methyl-2-pentanone	60	6.04	0.028	1.1	
5/6/2009	9	acetic acid	60	6.04	0.1	6.7	J
5/6/2009	9	α-pinene	60	6.04	0.48	14	J
5/6/2009	9	hexanal	60	6.04	0.073	2.9	J
5/6/2009	9	nonanal	60	6.04	0.18	5.1	J
5/6/2009	9	propanoic acid, 2-methyl	60	6.04	0.039	1.8	J
5/6/2009	9	tetradecane	60	6.04	0.062	1.3	J
5/6/2009	10	acetic acid	60	6.08	0.51	34	J
5/6/2009	10	α-pinene	60	6.08	0.46	14	J
5/6/2009	10	formic acid	60	6.08	0.055	4.8	J
5/6/2009	10	hexanal	60	6.08	0.097	3.8	J
5/6/2009	10	nonanal	60	6.08	0.22	6.2	J
5/6/2009	10	styrene	60	6.08	0.03	1.2	
5/6/2009	10	tetradecane	60	6.08	0.056	1.1	J
5/6/2009	11	acetic acid	60	6.05	0.69	46	J
5/6/2009	11	acetone	60	6.05	0.079	5.5	
5/6/2009	11	α-pinene	60	6.05	0.46	14	J
5/6/2009	11	hexanal	60	6.05	0.075	3.0	J
5/6/2009	11	nonanal	60	6.05	0.14	4.0	J
5/6/2009	11	propanoic acid, 2-methyl	60	6.05	0.059	2.7	J
5/6/2009	11	styrene	60	6.05	0.027	1.1	
5/6/2009	11	tetradecane	60	6.05	0.065	1.3	J
5/6/2009	12	acetic acid	60	6.04	0.53	36	J
5/6/2009	12	α-pinene	60	6.04	0.25	7.4	J
5/6/2009	12	hexanal	60	6.04	0.056	2.2	J
5/6/2009	12	nonanal	60	6.04	0.11	3.1	J
5/6/2009	12	phenol	60	6.04	0.027	1.2	J
5/6/2009	12	styrene	60	6.04	0.03	1.2	
5/6/2009	12	tetradecane	60	6.04	0.054	1.1	J

Date	Trailer	Analyte	Sample Duration (minutes)	Sample Volume (liters)	Sample Mass (μg)	Concen-tration (ppb)	Qual-ifier
5/6/2009	13	nonanal	60	6.04	0.016	0.46	J
5/6/2009	14	acetic acid	60	6.05	0.61	41	J
5/6/2009	14	α-pinene	60	6.05	0.36	11	J
5/6/2009	14	formic acid	60	6.05	0.054	4.7	J
5/6/2009	14	hexanal	60	6.05	0.054	2.1	J
5/6/2009	14	nonanal	60	6.05	0.1	2.8	J
5/6/2009	14	propanoic acid, 2-methyl	60	6.05	0.097	4.5	J
5/6/2009	14	tetradecane	60	6.05	0.044	0.90	J
5/6/2009	15	acetone	60	6.04	0.034	2.4	
5/6/2009	15	α-pinene	60	6.04	0.41	12	J
5/6/2009	15	hexanal	60	6.04	0.087	3.5	J
5/6/2009	15	nonanal	60	6.04	0.11	3.1	J
5/6/2009	15	phenol	60	6.04	0.035	1.5	J
5/6/2009	15	propanoic acid, 2-methyl	60	6.04	0.056	2.6	J
5/6/2009	15	styrene	60	6.04	0.057	2.2	
5/6/2009	15	tetradecane	60	6.04	0.069	1.4	J
5/6/2009	16	acetic acid	60	6.05	0.038	2.6	J
5/6/2009	16	acetonitrile	60	6.05	0.021	2.1	J
5/6/2009	16	butane, 2-methyl-	60	6.05	0.028	1.6	J
5/6/2009	16	dichlorodifluormethane	60	6.05	0.094	3.1	
5/6/2009	16	nonanal	60	6.05	0.027	0.77	J
5/6/2009	17	acetic acid	0	0	0.37	N/A	J
5/6/2009	17	α-pinene	0	0	0.37	N/A	J
5/6/2009	17	hexanal	0	0	0.066	N/A	J
5/6/2009	17	nonanal	0	0	0.11	N/A	J
5/6/2009	17	propanoic acid, 2-methyl	0	0	0.073	N/A	J
5/6/2009	17	tetradecane	0	0	0.039	N/A	J
5/13/2009	1	acetic acid	60	5.94	0.41	28	J
5/13/2009	1	acetone	60	5.94	0.15	11	
5/13/2009	1	α-pinene	60	5.94	0.37	11	J
5/13/2009	1	dichlorodifluormethane	60	5.94	0.029	0.99	
5/13/2009	1	ethanol	60	5.94	0.032	2.9	
5/13/2009	1	hexanal	60	5.94	0.054	2.2	J
5/13/2009	1	methylene chloride	60	5.94	0.035	1.7	
5/13/2009	1	nonanal	60	5.94	0.11	3.2	J
5/13/2009	1	propanoic acid, 2-methyl	60	5.94	0.047	2.2	J
5/13/2009	1	styrene	60	5.94	0.03	1.2	
5/13/2009	1	tetradecane	60	5.94	0.055	1.1	J
5/13/2009	2	acetic acid	60	6.08	0.21	14	J
5/13/2009	2	acetone	60	6.08	0.053	3.7	
5/13/2009	2	α-pinene	60	6.08	0.24	7.1	J
5/13/2009	2	hexanal	60	6.08	0.059	2.3	J

Date	Trailer	Analyte	Sample Duration (minutes)	Sample Volume (liters)	Sample Mass (μg)	Concen-tration (ppb)	Qual-ifier
5/13/2009	2	nonanal	60	6.08	0.12	3.4	J
5/13/2009	2	propanoic acid, 2-methyl	60	6.08	0.032	1.5	J
5/13/2009	2	styrene	60	6.08	0.083	3.2	
5/13/2009	2	tetradecane	60	6.08	0.055	1.1	
5/13/2009	3	acetic acid	60	6.11	0.12	8.0	J
5/13/2009	3	acetone	60	6.11	0.08	5.5	
5/13/2009	3	α-pinene	60	6.11	0.26	7.6	J
5/13/2009	3	hexanal	60	6.11	0.036	1.4	J
5/13/2009	3	methylene chloride	60	6.11	0.048	2.3	
5/13/2009	3	nonanal	60	6.11	0.11	3.1	J
5/13/2009	3	propanoic acid, 2-methyl	60	6.11	0.026	1.2	J
5/13/2009	3	styrene	60	6.11	0.045	1.7	
5/13/2009	3	tetradecane	60	6.11	0.05	1.0	J
5/13/2009	4	acetic acid	60	6.07	0.4	27	J
5/13/2009	4	acetone	60	6.07	0.081	5.6	
5/13/2009	4	α-pinene	60	6.07	0.39	11.5	J
5/13/2009	4	hexanal	60	6.07	0.042	1.7	J
5/13/2009	4	methylene chloride	60	6.07	0.051	2.4	
5/13/2009	4	nonanal	60	6.07	0.1	2.8	J
5/13/2009	4	propanoic acid, 2-methyl	60	6.07	0.053	2.4	J
5/13/2009	4	styrene	60	6.07	0.043	1.7	
5/13/2009	4	tetradecane	60	6.07	0.06	1.2	J
5/13/2009	5	acetic acid	60	6.08	0.3	20	J
5/13/2009	5	acetone	60	6.08	0.13	9.0	
5/13/2009	5	α-pinene	60	6.08	0.5	15	J
5/13/2009	5	hexanal	60	6.08	0.073	2.9	J
5/13/2009	5	methylene chloride	60	6.08	0.06	2.8	
5/13/2009	5	nonanal	60	6.08	0.16	4.5	J
5/13/2009	5	propanoic acid, 2-methyl	60	6.08	0.057	2.6	J
5/13/2009	5	styrene	60	6.08	0.052	2.0	
5/13/2009	5	tetradecane	60	6.08	0.06	1.2	J
5/13/2009	6	acetic acid	60	6.08	0.28	19	J
5/13/2009	6	acetone	60	6.08	0.055	3.8	
5/13/2009	6	α-pinene	60	6.08	0.24	7.1	J
5/13/2009	6	hexanal	60	6.08	0.05	2.0	J
5/13/2009	6	methylene chloride	60	6.08	0.027	1.3	J
5/13/2009	6	nonanal	60	6.08	0.1	2.8	J
5/13/2009	6	propanoic acid, 2-methyl	60	6.08	0.026	1.2	J
5/13/2009	6	styrene	60	6.08	0.037	1.4	J
5/13/2009	6	tetradecane	60	6.08	0.058	1.2	J
5/13/2009	7	acetic acid	60	6.07	0.45	30	J
5/13/2009	7	acetone	60	6.07	0.12	8.3	

Date	Trailer	Analyte	Sample Duration (minutes)	Sample Volume (liters)	Sample Mass (μg)	Concen-tration (ppb)	Qual-ifier
5/13/2009	7	α-pinene	60	6.07	0.37	11	J
5/13/2009	7	dichlorodifluormethane	60	6.07	0.025	0.83	
5/13/2009	7	ethanol	60	6.07	0.036	3.2	
5/13/2009	7	hexanal	60	6.07	0.046	1.8	J
5/13/2009	7	methylene chloride	60	6.07	0.059	2.8	
5/13/2009	7	nonanal	60	6.07	0.11	3.1	J
5/13/2009	7	propanoic acid, 2-methyl	60	6.07	0.088	4.0	J
5/13/2009	7	styrene	60	6.07	0.067	2.6	
5/13/2009	7	tetradecane	60	6.07	0.084	1.7	J
5/13/2009	8	acetic acid	60	6.09	0.42	28	J
5/13/2009	8	α-pinene	60	6.09	0.3	8.8	J
5/13/2009	8	hexanal	60	6.09	0.073	2.9	J
5/13/2009	8	nonanal	60	6.09	0.17	4.8	J
5/13/2009	8	phenol	60	6.09	0.043	1.8	J
5/13/2009	8	propanoic acid, 2-methyl	60	6.09	0.058	2.6	J
5/13/2009	8	styrene	60	6.09	0.061	2.4	
5/13/2009	8	tetradecane	60	6.09	0.11	2.2	J
5/13/2009	9	acetic acid	60	6.08	0.43	29	J
5/13/2009	9	acetone	60	6.08	0.069	4.8	
5/13/2009	9	α-pinene	60	6.08	0.46	14	J
5/13/2009	9	ethanol	60	6.08	0.026	2.3	
5/13/2009	9	hexanal	60	6.08	0.063	2.5	J
5/13/2009	9	isopropyl alcohol	60	6.08	0.082	5.5	
5/13/2009	9	methylene chloride	60	6.08	0.29	14	
5/13/2009	9	nonanal	60	6.08	0.15	4.2	J
5/13/2009	9	propanoic acid, 2-methyl	60	6.08	0.053	2.4	J
5/13/2009	9	styrene	60	6.08	0.042	1.6	
5/13/2009	9	tetradecane	60	6.08	0.046	0.93	J
5/13/2009	10	acetic acid	60	6.07	0.1	6.7	J
5/13/2009	10	α-pinene	60	6.07	0.5	15	J
5/13/2009	10	ethanol	60	6.07	1.3	110	
5/13/2009	10	hexanal	60	6.07	0.056	2.2	J
5/13/2009	10	methylene chloride	60	6.07	0.25	12	
5/13/2009	10	nonanal	60	6.07	0.15	4.3	J
5/13/2009	10	propanoic acid, 2-methyl	60	6.07	0.044	2.0	J
5/13/2009	10	styrene	60	6.07	0.052	2.0	
5/13/2009	11	acetic acid	60	6.03	0.34	23	J
5/13/2009	11	acetone	60	6.03	0.1	7.0	
5/13/2009	11	α-pinene	60	6.03	0.48	14	J
5/13/2009	11	ethanol	60	6.03	0.027	2.4	
5/13/2009	11	hexanal	60	6.03	0.071	2.8	J
5/13/2009	11	isopropyl alcohol	60	6.03	0.037	2.5	

Date	Trailer	Analyte	Sample Duration (minutes)	Sample Volume (liters)	Sample Mass (µg)	Concen-tration (ppb)	Qual-ifier
5/13/2009	11	methylene chloride	60	6.03	0.34	16.2	
5/13/2009	11	nonanal	60	6.03	0.14	4.0	J
5/13/2009	11	propanoic acid, 2-methyl	60	6.03	0.052	2.4	J
5/13/2009	11	styrene	60	6.03	0.054	2.1	
5/13/2009	11	tetradecane	60	6.03	0.06	1.2	J
5/13/2009	12	acetic acid	60	6.04	0.23	16	J
5/13/2009	12	acetone	60	6.04	0.045	3.1	
5/13/2009	12	α-pinene	60	6.04	0.28	8.3	J
5/13/2009	12	hexanal	60	6.04	0.047	1.9	J
5/13/2009	12	isopropyl alcohol	60	6.04	0.061	4.1	
5/13/2009	12	methylene chloride	60	6.04	0.16	7.6	
5/13/2009	12	nonanal	60	6.04	0.12	3.4	J
5/13/2009	12	propanoic acid, 2-methyl	60	6.04	0.064	2.9	J
5/13/2009	12	tetradecane	60	6.04	0.068	1.4	J
5/13/2009	13	acetic acid	60	6.05	0.071	4.8	J
5/13/2009	13	α-pinene	60	6.05	0.44	13	J
5/13/2009	13	dichlorodifluormethane	60	6.05	0.043	1.4	
5/13/2009	13	ethanol	60	6.05	0.03	2.6	
5/13/2009	13	hexanal	60	6.05	0.061	2.4	J
5/13/2009	13	isopropyl alcohol	60	6.05	0.081	5.5	
5/13/2009	13	methylene chloride	60	6.05	0.5	24	
5/13/2009	13	nonanal	60	6.05	0.1	2.8	J
5/13/2009	13	propanoic acid, 2-methyl	60	6.05	0.039	1.8	J
5/13/2009	13	styrene	60	6.05	0.039	1.5	
5/13/2009	13	tetradecane	60	6.05	0.045	0.92	J
5/13/2009	14	acetic acid	60	6.05	0.35	24	J
5/13/2009	14	α-pinene	60	6.05	0.46	14	J
5/13/2009	14	hexanal	60	6.05	0.054	2.1	J
5/13/2009	14	methylene chloride	60	6.05	0.15	7.1	
5/13/2009	14	nonanal	60	6.05	0.11	3.1	J
5/13/2009	14	propanoic acid, 2-methyl	60	6.05	0.11	5.1	J
5/13/2009	14	styrene	60	6.05	0.043	1.7	
5/13/2009	14	tetradecane	60	6.05	0.057	1.2	J
5/13/2009	15	acetic acid	60	6.05	0.63	42	J
5/13/2009	15	acetone	60	6.05	0.11	7.7	
5/13/2009	15	α-pinene	60	6.05	0.53	16	J
5/13/2009	15	dichlorodifluormethane	60	6.05	0.043	1.4	
5/13/2009	15	ethanol	60	6.05	0.039	3.4	
5/13/2009	15	hexanal	60	6.05	0.067	2.7	J
5/13/2009	15	isopropyl alcohol	60	6.05	0.11	7.4	
5/13/2009	15	methylene chloride	60	6.05	0.51	24	
5/13/2009	15	nonanal	60	6.05	0.12	3.4	J

Date	Trailer	Analyte	Sample Duration (minutes)	Sample Volume (liters)	Sample Mass (μg)	Concen-tration (ppb)	Qual-ifier
5/13/2009	15	propanoic acid, 2-methyl	60	6.05	0.072	3.3	J
5/13/2009	15	styrene	60	6.05	0.11	4.3	
5/13/2009	15	tetradecane	60	6.05	0.05	1.0	J
5/13/2009	16	acetic acid	60	6.04	0.043	2.9	J
5/13/2009	16	acetonitrile	60	6.04	0.16	16	J
5/13/2009	16	dichlorodifluormethane	60	6.04	0.028	0.94	
5/13/2009	16	ethanol	60	6.04	0.041	3.6	
5/13/2009	16	isopropyl alcohol	60	6.04	0.12	8.1	
5/13/2009	16	methylene chloride	60	6.04	0.7	33	
5/13/2009	16	nonanal	60	6.04	0.029	0.83	J
5/13/2009	17	ethanol	0	0	0.035	N/A	
5/13/2009	17	isopropyl alcohol	0	0	0.042	N/A	
5/13/2009	17	methylene chloride	0	0	0.4	N/A	
5/13/2009	17	nonanal	0	0	0.023	N/A	J

www.ingramcontent.com/pod-product-compliance
Lightning Source LLC
Chambersburg PA
CBHW080246180526
45167CB00006B/2436